The Bra Book

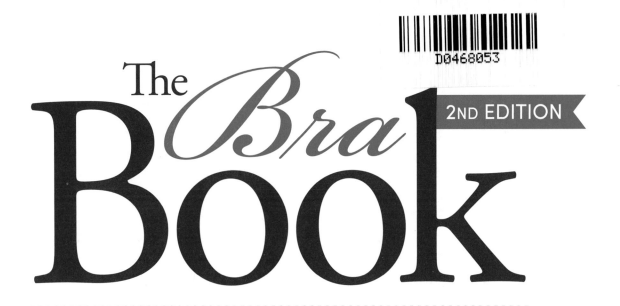

2ND EDITION

An Intimate Guide to Finding the Right Bra,
Shapewear, Swimsuit, and More!

JENÉ LUCIANI

Illustrations by Ralph Voltz

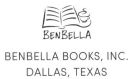

BENBELLA

BENBELLA BOOKS, INC.
DALLAS, TEXAS

BenBella Books, Inc.
10440 N. Central Expressway, Suite 800
Dallas, TX 75231
www.benbellabooks.com
Send feedback to feedback@benbellabooks.com

Printed in United States of America
10 9 8 7 6 5 4 3 2 1

Library of Congress Cataloging-in-Publication Data
Names: Luciani, Jene, author.
Title: The bra book : an intimate guide to finding the right bra, shapewear, swimsuit, and more! / Jene Luciani ; illustrations by Ralph Voltz.
Description: Second edition. | Dallas, Texas : BenBella Books, 2017. Includes bibliographical references and index.
Identifiers: LCCN 2016049060 (print) | LCCN 2016049683 (ebook) | ISBN 9781944648329 (paperback) | ISBN 9781944648398 (electronic)
Subjects: LCSH: Brassieres. | Sleepwear. | Bathing suits. | Clothing and dress measurements. | BISAC: HEALTH & FITNESS / Beauty & Grooming.
Classification: LCC TT677 .L83 2017 (print) | LCC TT677 (ebook) | DDC 687/.22—dc23
LC record available at https://lccn.loc.gov/2016049060

Distributed by Perseus Distribution
www.perseusdistribution.com
To place orders through Perseus Distribution:
Tel: (800) 343-4499 | *Fax:* (800) 351-5073
E-mail: orderentry@perseusbooks.com

Proofreading by Kim Broderick
Cover and text design and composition by Kit Sweeney
Printed by Versa Press

This book is dedicated to all the women out there who are taking the time to read this book and be the best they can be, in the skin they're in!

To my family, Patrick, GiGi, Ayva, Hammy, and Kalen: love you more than life.

And to my mom, who has "supported" me from the start.

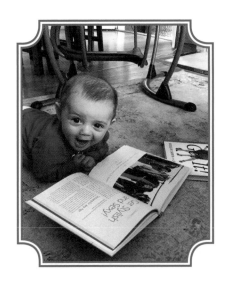
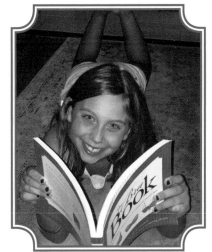

CONTENTS

ACKNOWLEDGMENTS

· ·

FIRST, THANKS TO ALL OF YOU WHO HAVE supported me on this journey since the first edition of *The Bra Book* was published in 2009! From becoming Dr. Oz's "bra guru" to meeting Oprah and getting her nod of approval, it has exceeded my wildest dreams—and all because I am passionate about sharing what I've learned over the years on this topic with all of you!

Extra special thanks to Michael Ebeling, my illustrious literary agent, and my talent agent Mark Turner, for always believing in me and my work. To my "family" at BenBella Books, especially Glenn Yeffeth, who was enthusiastic about this project from the start, and is giving it a second go-round! My editor Leah Wilson deserves as much credit for this book as I do, and is now a "bra guru" in her own right.

To my fellow journalists and members of the media, especially Joanne, Kathie, Hoda, and the gang over at NBC's *TODAY*, many thanks for your continued support.

To Gigi, who was in my belly while I was writing this book the first time around, and Kalen, who was there for the second go-round, both of whom I cannot thank enough for the extra huge (albeit temporary) increases in my bra size (we're talking G cups, people!) and first-hand experience of how pregnancy can royally mess with your boobies!

To my partner Patrick, his children Ayva and Patrick, and to my parents, siblings, and extended family and friends, I know cup sizes and band measurements are probably not the most interesting topic to you but thank you for embracing my life's passion and work and for always "supporting" me.

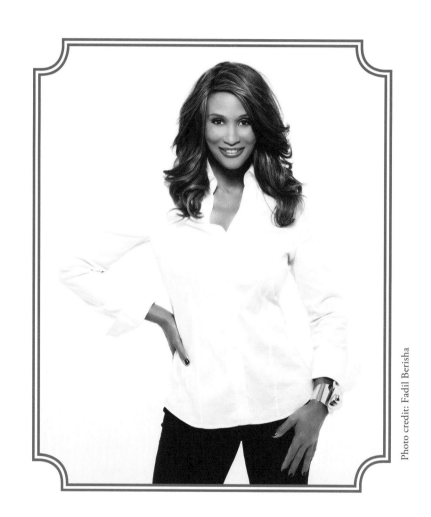

A LETTER FROM BEVERLY JOHNSON

Dear Readers of *The Bra Book*:

As I'm writing this, it's been more than thirty-five years since I first graced the cover of *Vogue* magazine—the first African American model to do so. People say that I am the first black supermodel, which is something I am very proud of. As I look back on my career, I think about what I have gone through as far as body image in an industry that's really all about what you look like on the outside. As a model and actress, as well as a mom, entrepreneur, author, activist, and athlete, I am conscious every day about staying healthy and fit and embracing my body. It's an ongoing process. Like most women, it took me many years to feel comfortable in my own skin.

Growing up in a small town near Buffalo, New York, I was a competitive swimmer, so my body was a vessel for my sport. I wasn't self-conscious about it but I wasn't really conscious of it, either. It was just *there*. Though I was teased by my brother about being "flat as an ironing board," I never internalized it. But I was jealous of my younger sister because she was more "developed" than I was. It seemed the boys were always after her.

It wasn't until I became a model and my body was celebrated that I began to think about my breasts. To be honest, it was mostly because I had this dream of becoming a lingerie model. They made double to triple the day rate of us regular models. Those ladies in the Sears catalogs modeling bras and panties made tons of money and I wanted that, too! They didn't even need to have big portfolios, just a little bit of cleavage. They were the equivalent of the Victoria's Secret girls of today. In modeling, it was big business. I kept asking my agency to book me for those jobs but I always got the same answer: "You don't have a lingerie body." It finally dawned on me what I was lacking—ample breasts. In the '80s, I had tried this "Thighmaster"-looking thing that you squashed together with your hands to increase your bust size. All the models had this. Every night, I used it fifteen times. Needless to say, it didn't work.

I let go of those dreams and continued to enjoy a successful career in modeling, with more than 500 magazine covers to my credit. For high-fashion and editorial work, they wanted you to look like a "human hanger," which is still the case today, so having boobs was frowned upon. I once overheard a designer say about another model, "Oh, she has these horrible breasts. They are messing up my design; I can't hire her with those big things!" My small stature worked for me.

Whether you are big- or small-busted, this book will educate you not only about bras and your breasts, but how to feel good about what God has given you and how to forever be at peace with your breasts. While many of us curse uncomfortable bras or the appearance of our breasts, what you will read throughout these chapters will teach you how to embrace what you have—and work with it. I wish I'd had a guide like this when I was "growing up" in the fashion industry. No one was there to tell me that what I had was okay, and I always envied others who had what I felt I lacked.

I have learned many lessons over the years, and many have been through trial and error. But one thing I know is that if you feel good about your body, and educate yourself on how to make the most of what you have, you can't go wrong. Whether it's a bra that makes you feel like you have more than you do, or a bra that makes you feel "whole" again after a life-changing mastectomy, it truly can be life-changing when you find the right one. Bras have certainly come a long way since their invention, and in my eyes, so have I. I wish you all the same in your journeys.

XOXO,
Beverly Johnson

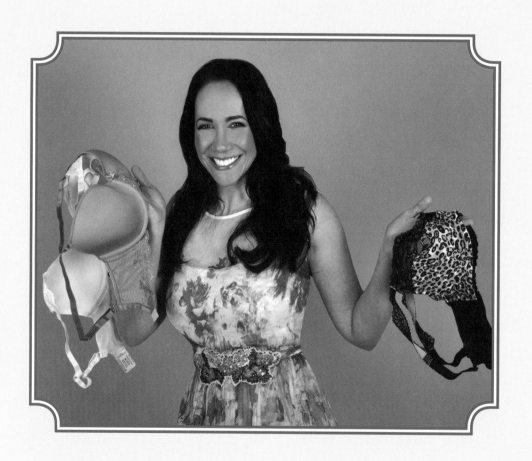

INTRODUCTION

Dᴜʀɪɴɢ ᴍʏ 2004 ᴡᴇᴅᴅɪɴɢ ʀᴇᴄᴇᴘᴛɪᴏɴ, my best friend Melissa stood up to give a speech that, several years and one divorce later, is still fresh in my mind. She began with this: "As long as I've known Jené, she has always been searching for the perfect 'one.' The perfect man, the perfect job, the perfect hair color." Naturally, she garnered a laugh from the crowd. What she said also really resonated with me, but there was one important thing missing from that list.

As women, we are also on a constant quest to find the perfect bra. While some of us simply complain about never being able to find "the right one," others just give up entirely, because the quest for the Perfect Bra—the bra that makes her both look good *and* feel good—seems endless. Sadly, it's not as simple as just walking into a store. And women are afraid to ask for help, or simply don't know the right questions to ask. So unsurprisingly, when it came to writing THE essential guide on all things bras, most women I spoke to said, "Why didn't anyone think of this before?!"

In the nearly forty years of my life, and especially in the eight years since the first edition of *The Bra Book* came out, I've seen bras put women through a range of emotions: denial ("But I'm a size 34C!"), anger ("My bra is SO uncomfortable!"), frustration ("I just can't seem to find one that FITS!"), sadness ("I've now had to switch to a bra that LIFTS!") . . . well, you get the picture. Some just plain give up. And I always wondered: Why wasn't anyone helping us? Why wasn't anyone out there clearing up our confusion about the sizing system, or even just offering basic information about this undergarment that's so essential to our lives?

There are many reasons we all care so much about bras. A good one makes us feel good inside and out. It supports us, even protects us, concealing our flaws and highlighting our strengths. The right one can make us feel confident and sexy—like a woman should!

The bra's ability to change the way we see our breasts, and how that can make us feel, is more important than it sounds. Women in society are often identified—and even judged—by their breasts. Just ask Dolly Parton or Pamela Anderson. And so we tend to judge ourselves by them, too.

My own breasts have undergone many changes. I developed during puberty with a deformity called Tubular Breast Syndrome, which caused my breasts to be completely lopsided: one breast was a full cup size smaller than the other and had a "tube-like" shape. After many traumatic years trying to hide and mask my deformity through the use of bras with removable pads, I decided to undergo a breast reconstruction.

Two surgeries later, my breasts "appeared" normal under my clothes, but I was unable to breastfeed either of my children as I would have liked, as my milk ducts were damaged and I only got milk in one breast.

I'm sure you can relate in some shape or form, whether you have some type of breast deformity as I did, or just because you've simply watched your breasts change after childbirth, from breastfeeding, or with age.

As women, we are much harder on ourselves than we should be. How our breasts look and feel has the power, for good or for ill, to change how *we* look and feel. And bras are a big part of that. Wearing the right bra can provide a much-needed "boost," both in confidence and otherwise. As in my case for all those years, they can even make you simply feel "normal." It's a powerful little piece of fabric!

My goal with this book is to educate and, I hope, empower you. While the bra is now a centenarian, its hundred-year presence in our wardrobes doesn't change the fact that many of us still feel we are venturing into unknown territory. Oprah helped make us aware, when she declared that America needed a Bra Intervention. On her talk show, Tyra Banks actually held a *bra burning*, showing exactly how frustrated, sad, and angered we are by our bras. The reason? We don't understand them—and until now there hasn't been a place where all the information we need was accurately and succinctly pulled together so that we finally could. *The Bra Book* takes away the mystery by showing you not only how your bra works, but how to make it work for *you*.

I've been fortunate enough to be part of the charge leading the cause to help women learn how to love their "girls" and keep them properly supported. In the years since I first wrote *The Bra Book*, I've become Dr. Oz's "Bra Guru," appearing on many episodes giving advice to millions of viewers. I've also given bra fit tips and advice on talk shows like *Bethenny*, *The Meredith Vieira Show*, and

Bra Book Buzz

"Everyone needs this book!"
– Kathie Lee Gifford, to viewers of *Today*

"Jené is, to me, one of the most important guests we've had on this show."
– Wendy Williams

"Thank God Jené's here!"
– Ricki Lake

The Ricki Lake Show, and regularly give bra, beauty, and style advice on NBC's *TODAY*. My advice has appeared in national magazines including *Marie Claire*, *Cosmopolitan*, *First for Women*, and *Woman's World*. I even had the chance to meet Oprah herself, the woman who first got everyone buzzing about bras again, and show her *The Bra Book*. She told me she was glad I wrote it because the topic was "so important" for women. What better endorsement could an author ask for then a positive remark from Oprah herself?

I knew it was a risk, writing *The Bra Book*. Would women take it seriously? And prior to me hitting the talk show circuit, most of the "experts" you saw on TV talking about bras were *selling* them. As a fashion journalist and style expert, my mission is and always has been to educate women and to do the legwork so you don't have to. You don't have to spend a lot of money to look and feel great in the skin you're in and to love the boobs you've got!

Whether you have embraced your breasts your entire life or been adversely affected by them in some way, as I have, this book will give you the support you need—in more ways than one. Just like your best girlfriend or your mom, this book

will, I hope, be a comforting voice on your journey to feeling confident in your skin *and* your bra. The only emotion your bra should evoke is happiness—and after *The Bra Book*, it will be.

For this second edition, I've added entirely new sections—one on swimwear, because so many women don't realize that they can find perfect fitting swimwear, based on their bra size, and one on shapewear, since these days, what's underneath is not just about the bra.

Do you need any more reason to turn the page than that?

Don't forget to share what you've learned with all the other women in your life who could use a little "boost," too! Moms, sisters, girlfriends, co-workers . . .
especially new moms and those who have gone through a major life change that affected their breasts, such as a battle with breast cancer. Spread the knowledge and positive message. Let's all get educated together!

one

The Herstory
of
Bras

Every woman has a "herstory." Some of it she'd like to remember, and some of it she'd rather forget. But when it comes to a woman's herstory with bras, there are often many memorable moments.

No matter how old we get, we often still remember our major bra milestones. Remember when Mom or Dad took you to the local department store to buy your very first training bra (even though you most likely had nothing to go in it)? Or how about when you realized that a little padding goes a long way?

"The bra is with us through every stage of life," says Mara Susskind Kalcheim, an intimate apparel industry expert who has been in the business for more than forty years. "As a young girl, you are dying for your first bra. As a young woman, you want a sexy bra to wear for your first boyfriend and something that will support developing breasts. As you grow into motherhood, you need a maternity bra and bras that will fit your changing figure. In your thirties and forties, [you need] something more steady and supportive but still sexy, and then as you get older, you go for comfort!"

While it's no doubt the bra has left a large imprint on our personal pasts, that little piece of fabric with the molded cups and many clever pseudonyms ("over-the-shoulder boulder holder," "brassiere," "hooter hoister") has left many a mark on our society as well! Like reporter Samantha Thompson Smith says in her 2007 article for McClatchy Newspapers: "Love it, hate it, burn it, or embrace it, the bra endures!" Over the years the bra has even become a fashion icon in its own right.

Before you can learn about all the bra has to offer, it's important to understand how the bra came to be. Here is a mostly factual, if somewhat tongue-in-cheek, roundup of some of the highlights of the century long herstory of the bra:

The Herstory of Bras

▶ 1907: French couturier Paul Poiret loosens up the corset (a binding garment used for centuries to cinch the waist and support the breasts) and makes the first "brassiere." *Vogue* magazine coins the term.

16

▼ 1913: The bra as we know it is born when socialite Mary Phelps Jacob fashions together two hankies with some pink ribbon and cord. Friends encourage her to patent her design and a year later she sells it to Warner Brothers Corset Company.[1]

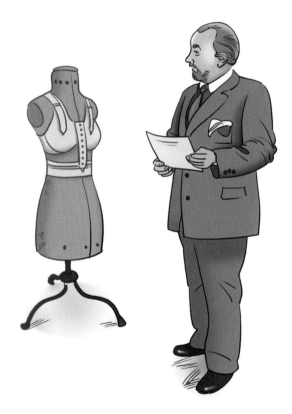

1917: The U.S. enters World War I and women are asked to stop wearing corsets to conserve steel. Some 28,000 tons

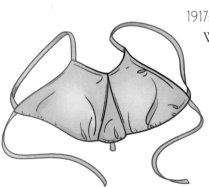

1. While Jacob is perhaps the most well-known bra creator in history, many others would claim *they* actually "invented" the bra, including Maidenform founder Ida Rosenthal.

are diverted, enough to build an entire battleship.

▶ 1920s: Binding "flapper bras" are all the rage. Flat chests are in and big busts are taboo.

▶ (far right) 1930s: Advertisements aren't allowed to show photographs of women in bras so savvy companies use drawings of models instead!

1935: Cleavage starts to make a comeback. Founders of Maidenform Co. introduce "cup sizes" from A to D.[2]

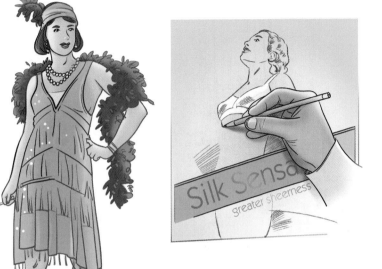

Silk Sensa...
greater sheerness

For the first time, "getting an A" is considered a bad thing.

1939: The word "bra" is officially added to the English dictionary

17

BRA HERSTORY FACT

Rome wasn't built in a day and neither was the bra. Did you know some say the bra dates all the way back to 2000 B.C.? This early corset-style bra was open at the front to the waist, leaving the breasts uncovered. Small strips of leather curved around the outline of the breasts for support.

2. Although there are conflicting reports on the date Maidenform actually began selling these different cup sizes, some say it was as early as 1922!

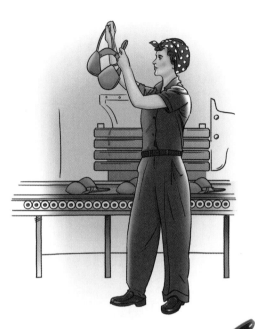

▼ (bottom) 1947: Kleenex sales plummet when Frederick's of Hollywood unveils the world's first padded bra and, a year later, the push-up bra. Boys everywhere rejoice.

◀ 1950s: Missile or "bullet-shaped" bras that create a pointed appearance under sweaters gain prevalence. Hollywood's A-list actresses, including Jayne Mansfield, capitalize on the trend.

1951: Wrapture's blow-up bra leaves wearers breathless when they have to inflate their own cups using an attached straw. "We must, we must, we must increase our bust" becomes the mantra for a generation, and women everywhere begin exercising their chest muscles in hopes of increasing their, er, size.

1958: DuPont introduces Lycra, a fiber that can stretch significantly while still retaining its shape, allowing

18

(although "brassiere" has been in the Oxford dictionary since 1912). Little did we know "bootylicious" would follow suit just a few decades later.

▲ 1941: World War II brings a shortage of the metals and other materials used to make bras and corsets, so synthetic fibers like nylon are used as an alternative.

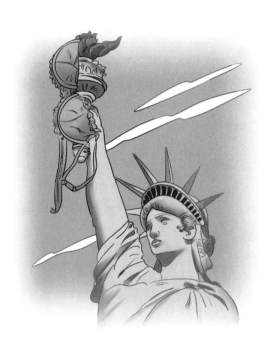

bras, although none are ever confirmed to have actually been on fire.

1969: A woman in San Francisco publically removes her bra during "Anti-Bra Day," a day to protest the pressures society puts on women.

That same year, the medical community warns women of the adverse effects of going braless.

1977: Athletic gals finally get some support, too, when the Jogbra is introduced. The world's first "sports bra" consists of two male jockstraps, sewn together (yikes!).

1983: The Material Girl shows the world less "material" is more. Madonna shocks fans (but cements her place in fashion history) by wearing her bra as a top while promoting her debut

19

corsets and bras to be more lightweight, comfortable, and breathable. Gals everywhere breathe a sigh of bra-lief!

▲ 1968: The bra—or lack thereof—becomes an icon of American history and a symbol of feminism when protestors hurl their bras into trashcans during the Miss America pageant in Atlantic City. Media reports claim the pro-women's liberation crowd is burning the

BRA HERSTORY FACT

A *Time* magazine article dating to 1965 cites the average price of bras at just $4.

album. It won't be the only time Madonna makes news in a bra.

1985: Perhaps a nod to the growing popularity of breast augmentation, manufacturers start offering sizes above a DD.

▼ 1986: Frederick's of Hollywood opens the country's first "Bra Museum," housing lingerie worn by celebrities from the previous four decades. The museum garners national attention just six years later when it is looted during the Los Angeles riots. Looters reportedly snatch a pair of Ava Gardner's "bloomers," among other items.

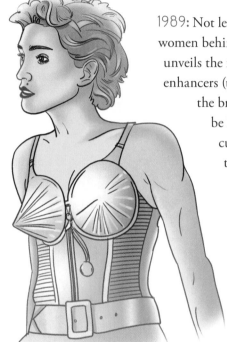

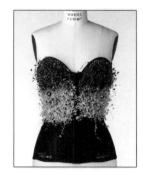

A corset designed by Diana Ross currently housed in Frederick's of Hollywood's flagship store, the site of the former museum.

1989: Not leaving smaller-busted women behind, Frederick's unveils the first silicone breast enhancers (they get placed inside the bra), which come to be known as "chicken cutlets." They become the first "food" ever embraced by Hollywood starlets.

◄ 1990: The bra hits a high "point" when Madonna's highly controversial cone-shaped style stuns folks in cities all across America during her Blonde Ambition World Tour. People everywhere are warned, "Kids, don't try these at home. They'll put your eye out!"

That same year, a Japanese company develops the world's largest bra. It has an under-bust measurement of 78'8", and a bust measurement of 91'10", according to *The Guinness Book of World Records*.

BRA HERSTORY FACT

Although breasts come in all shapes and sizes, the "ideal" shape of a woman's bosoms under her blouse is dictated by what's popular in society at the time. In the 1920s women flattened their breasts, and just a few decades later wore bras to make them look pointier. In the twenty-first century, women have been going under the knife to attain the roundest breasts possible.

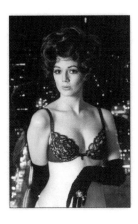

◄ 1994: "Hello, boys." The Wonderbra, a plunging push-up bra, goes on sale in the U.S. and chaos ensues. The company claims one is sold every fifteen seconds.

1995: Men get their first bra, if only on television. On an episode of the hit show *Seinfeld*, Kramer and Frank Costanza hatch a plan to sell a Velcro-fastened bra for men, but can't decide whether to call it the "bro" or the "mansiere."

▼ 1997: Fashion Forms introduces the Original Water Bra, a bra filled with water and oil (to keep the water from evaporating) that revolutionizes the push-up bra industry. It makes headlines when David Letterman tries to run over one with a truck and Jennifer Aniston reportedly has hers attacked by a chopstick.

1998: Tara Cavosie of Albany, New York, creates and patents the first "backless strapless bra." Department stores and retailers like Victoria's Secret quickly scoop it up. Clearly filling a consumer need, it flies off store shelves.

21

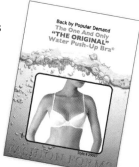

Back by Popular Demand
The One And Only
"THE ORIGINAL"
Water Push-Up Bra

1999: The Water Bra gets another fifteen minutes of fame on an episode of the sitcom *Will and Grace*. Debra Messing's character, Grace, wears the bra, only to have it "spring a leak" during an evening out. The Water Bra has since gone the way of the waterbed as a fad that has seemed to fizzle out, although it is still available for purchase online.

2004: Singer Janet Jackson sends censors into a flurry when, braless, she reveals a nipple during a Super Bowl performance on national television. The incident is attributed to a "wardrobe malfunction."

2005: Supermodel Karolina Kurkova sets tongues wagging in a $13 million diamond bra on the Victoria's Secret runway.

◄2006: The daytime talk show queens get everyone talking about bras! *The Oprah Winfrey Show* holds a "Bra Intervention." Oprah, known for covering "of the moment" topics and hot-button issues, declares: "America, you are wearing the wrong bra," and counts herself among the 85 percent of women believed to be incorrectly underclothed. A media blitz on the topic ensues. Supermodel turned talk-show diva Tyra Banks follows suit, devoting an episode of *The Tyra Banks Show* to throwing

BRA HERSTORY FACT

Us gals are growing. Published reports say that, in the last twenty years, the most popular bra size has increased from a 34B to a 36C!

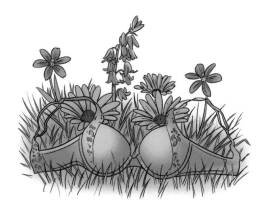

an on-set "panty party" and teaching viewers how to find properly fitting undergarments.

Due to what comes to be known as the "Oprah Winfrey Effect," bra sales go up 15 percent the following year, to $5.7 billion, according to the NPD Group, a research firm in Port Washington, New York.

▲ 2007: The bra turns 100 and continues to change with the times. In line with growing concern over the global warming crisis, the bra goes green when manufacturers start making bras using eco-friendly fabrics like bamboo blends.

▶ 2009: Women's perceptions of bra sizes are changing! An article cites DD as "the new C" as more and more women get fitted and learn their true sizes. Retailers

respond with offerings like larger cup sizes and more size combinations.

That same year, *The Bra Book* is published. Women everywhere finally have a guide to the world's most confusing undergarment!

▶ 2011: Yours truly makes waves in the fashion world by wearing the first dress made entirely out of bras in an appearance on *Project Runway*–famed designer Chris March's Bravo television show *Mad Fashion*. March used

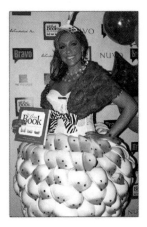

more than 200 bras for the project, which was subsequently featured in *Star* magazine's "Worst Dressed" list (oops!).

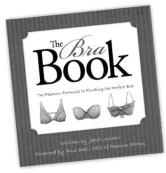

2013: A French researcher stirs up controversy when he releases a fifteen-year study of 300 women aged eighteen to thirty-five that shows wearing a bra over time actually *causes* sagging, not prevents it. (More on what

23

actually causes sagging, and what you can do to prevent it, in chapter 6.)

2014: The "Free the Nipple" campaign (#FreetheNipple) is launched to promote gender equality, and celebs like Lena Dunham,

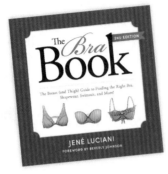

Scout Willis, and Kendell Jenner all go topless to support the cause.

2016: The sports bra gets a high-tech upgrade with the invention of the OMbra, which measures heart rate and distance and sends them to an iPhone app.

◄ 2017: The second edition of *The Bra Book* is released!

Remember when you learned your ABCs? Continue on to Chapter 2, where you'll learn them all over again—the ABCs of bras!

two

The ABCs
of
Bras

CHANCES ARE, IF YOU'RE OLD ENOUGH TO READ THIS BOOK, THEN YOU KNOW by now that the letters of the alphabet also correlate to the cup sizes of bras. Cup sizes range from AA to JJ and are anything but consistent—in fact, despite there *theoretically* being a standard for sizing, it can vary from vendor to vendor.

But there's a lot more to the "ABCs" of bras then just figuring out the cup sizing system. With more than forty separate components, a bra has enough engineering to make NASA envious! In fact, in an interview on NBC's *Today* show, Maidenform executive Manette Scheininger compared the bra to a suspension bridge, saying, "a bra and a bridge have to support and they have to be flexible. So a bra has to support the weight of the breast but it has to be flexible enough to move with the body because you want to be comfortable. And a bridge has to be supportive for the cars moving across it, but again, it has to be flexible for wind conditions and just the movement of the cars."

Luckily you don't need a degree in physics to get the basics of how your bra works. Understanding your bra can be as simple as A-B-C.

ANATOMY, BIOMECHANICS, AND PHYSICS: THE SCIENCE OF BRAS

While our bras do many things for us—shape our breasts, create a smooth line under clothing, and boost our confidence—the garment's most important job is providing support.

So how exactly do bras do this? It really comes down to basic physics. Think of the breast as a weight. Gravity pulls it down, and bras are designed to counteract that pull. Breast tissue is supported naturally by our chest muscles, skin, and ligaments—but they alone aren't enough to fight off the effects of gravity. Our bras do what our bodies alone cannot.

Some researchers say bras have only recently become a "science." A 2007 study at the University of Portsmouth in England looked at a bra's design and what it's doing for our bodies. In an article on the website LiveScience, the study's author Joanna Scurr is quoted as saying that, previously in bra design, "there was no research. It's like designing a car or kitchen equipment without first thinking 'what is the purpose of this?'"

The lack of research could be in part because the anatomy of our breasts is something of a puzzle. A woman's breasts can range from 10 ounces all the way up to 20 pounds or more in weight, and there is no definitive rhyme or reason to their structure. They are mostly made up of lobes and a network of ducts designed to produce milk. The rest of the breast is fat, tissue, and skin. Why exactly our breasts sag is a mystery, too. While many anatomists believe the connective breast tissue known as Cooper's ligaments provides our breasts' main support, others feel the skin plays the most important role in holding our breasts in place. Unfortunately, there are no definitive answers.

Scientists are also still trying to figure out exactly how our breasts move, and how a bra can best counteract that motion. In 2007, a group of biomechanists in Australia did a study on breast movement where they fitted seventy subjects with specially designed bras. According to a 2005 article in *Discover* magazine, they placed sensors under the straps to measure how much pressure was placed on the shoulders. They also placed electrodes on the subjects' torsos and necks to monitor muscle activity and LEDs on their sternums and nipples, and on

the bra's straps, to measure breast and torso movements. While the women all walked, jogged, and ran, the scientists were able to track their breasts' pattern of movement (it resembled a figure eight), how much their breasts moved, and how that movement was affected by wearing the bra. Obviously, larger breasts moved much more than the smaller breasts—although tests found that even A-cups move up to an average of 40mm (that's just under two inches, or about the length of a large paperclip) from their natural resting place. A 2007 British study found that breasts move in three directions during exercise: up and down, side to side, and forward and back. And while no one really knows for sure the long-term implications of such breast movements, it's presumed that they can cause breast pain and are the most likely reason for sagging.

What all these studies have confirmed is that the larger the breasts, the more they move. And the more breasts move, the more momentum they have. A well-designed bra stops that momentum. How? Let's take a look at the working parts of the bra, and the way they work together to give you the best possible support.

29

The Parts *of the* Bra

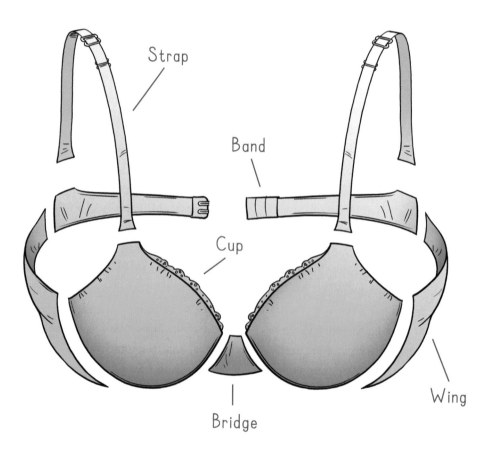

Strap

Band

Cup

Wing

Bridge

Simply Strapping: The straps are the parts of the bra that loop over your shoulders. Bra straps offer support but not primarily by holding the breasts up. Instead, they support the breasts by stabilizing them. They are also one of the few adjustable parts of the bra.

In that 2005 breast movement study, scientists found that the straps bear the brunt of the load generated by momentum during physical activity. And while the straps are obviously important for support, they shouldn't bear the *entire* burden. In a well-designed bra the straps only *help* with the heavy lifting. You'll know they are being overworked if they are digging into your shoulders and causing you discomfort.

To get the most support out of your bra straps, keep them on the tightest setting possible that does not cause you pain or discomfort. *Tip:* Start by making the straps as tight as possible and then loosen them up from there. Don't forget to tighten your straps each and every time you put your bra on!

I'm with the Band: The band is the part of the bra that wraps around the ribcage just below the breasts. The band is the most

> ### THE ABCs OF BRAS FAST FACT
> Hate having to readjust your bra straps every time you wear or wash your bra? It could be worse—your grandmother just had to put up with straps that were too loose. Adjusting your bra straps wasn't even an option until the 1940s!

31

important element of support because it holds the bra's cups (and the breast tissue within them) in place.

You can look at the bra like a teeter-totter—the more the band rides up in the back, the more the cups will come down in the front. Because of this, the band should fit snugly (but not too snugly; you should be able to fit one or two fingers underneath it) and lay completely level across your back. If it's too loose, it will ride up your back, allowing your breasts to sag.

She's Got Wings: The wings are the parts of the bra band that stretch from the side of the cup around the back to the place the band fastens. The wings provide most of the cup support by counterbalancing the weight of the breasts in front.

Captivating Cups: The cups are the parts of the bra that hold the breast tissue in place and act as the breasts' main means of support. They can also help to push breasts up and inward, creating cleavage.

Properly fitted cups should provide enough support to prevent the straps from digging into your shoulders. A cup with underwire is the most supportive—it allows the breasts' weight to be more evenly distributed to the straps and around the band.

Bridging the Gap: The bridge is the small piece of fabric located between the bra's cups. It may be a tiny piece of your overall bra, but it is actually an important part of proper support because it holds the cups at the front of the body, preventing the breasts from moving too far to either side. The bridge should fit completely flush against the body. If the bridge doesn't sit flat, your breasts will be pulled off to the side or the bra cups may ride up the undersides of your breasts.

Look at your bra like a puzzle—it's only complete (and properly supportive!) when all the "pieces" are put together properly. If they aren't, then your bra will not be doing its job—which could lead to discomfort in the present, and sagging in the future.

Getting to Know Your Bra

from A *to* Z

There's more to understanding bras than just knowing their working parts. Bras today come in all kinds of styles and all kinds of fabrics. Now that you know how the bra works, you need to understand the jargon that describes all the different bras available to you (and other important terms related to the bra).

The next few pages teach you all this information the old-fashioned way: with a bra alphabet!

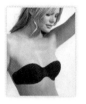

A

Adhesive or Backless Strapless Bra: A bra that lacks straps and a back band and is held up by medical-grade adhesive.

B

Balconette (or Balconet) Bra: A bra that covers only the lower three-quarters of the breasts. Unlike a demi cup, which is slanted, the tops of the cups are usually cut in a straight line across each breast.

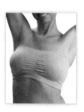

Bandeau Bra: A band of fabric that covers the breasts. It's usually stretchy and without straps, but sometimes has built-in cups.

Bra: When you look up bra in the dictionary, you are referred to the definition for brassiere, which according to Merriam-Webster is a noun for "a woman's undergarment to cover and support the breasts."

Bralette: A soft bra that has no underwire or structured cups. It resembles a camisole but instead of covering the midsection stops just short of the tummy with an elastic band.

Breast Petal: A small adhesive nipple cover that prevents the nipple from protruding under sheer garments.

Bustier: A bra that extends down over the midsection and usually has boning (small vertical support tubes made of metal or plastic) designed to push up the breasts. It's often worn under a wedding gown and resembles a corset.

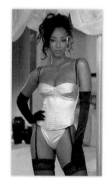

C

Cleavage: The effect attained by pushing two breasts together to create a vertical line down the middle.

34

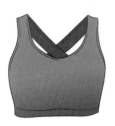

Compression Bra: A sports bra that presses (or *compresses*) breast tissue against the body to restrict its movement during exercise or other activity.

Contour Bra: A bra with lined or padded cups that hold their shape even when not being worn. According to lingerie reference intimateguide.com, the bra "offers significant coverage, a smooth shape, and hides the nipples—even under tight clothing."

Convertible Bra: A bra that can be worn multiple ways through the use of detachable straps. For example, you can wear it with a strap over each shoulder like a normal bra, but you can also take one strap off and wrap the other around your neck and hook it in the front to turn it into a halter bra. The convertible bra is versatile and can be adjusted to remain invisible under almost any neckline.

Corset-Style Bra: A bra designed to have the same aesthetic as the corset, a garment that was once worn to mold the

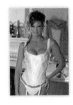

torso into a desired shape, but without the painful waist-whittling. They also push up the bust, much like a bustier.

Cotton: A natural fiber that is used to make many bras, especially those intended primarily for comfort. Cotton textiles are soft, cozy, fine, and breathable. They absorb moisture and are easy to wear and care for. According to atlastbras.com, the online home of Sacramento, California, store At Last . . . Bras and Lingerie, "Different qualities in cotton are dictated by how long and how fine the fiber is spun. The longer and finer the fiber is, the more valuable cotton becomes" (and the better the quality of the bra).

Cutlet: A gel pad that is made to be inserted inside a bra, under the breast tissue, to create a fuller look or boost up the breast. It is called a cutlet because of its not-so-subtle resemblance to actual chicken cutlets.

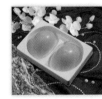

Cookie: No, not the kind you eat. This is the oval-shaped removable fabric pad usually

35

found in push-up bras. It does basically the same thing as a cutlet, but isn't as "natural" in look or feel.

Demi (or Demi-Cup) Bra:
A bra that covers the lower three-quarters of the breast and is great for pushing up breast tissue and creating cleavage.

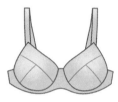

Double-Sided Tape: An adhesive tape that is coated with adhesive on both sides. It is designed to stick two lightweight surfaces together and can be used to hold a bra in place beneath a dress or top.

36

Encapsulation Bra:
A sports bra that has a separate cup for each breast (unlike the compression sports bra, where the breasts are treated as one mass).

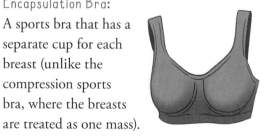

Front-Close Bra: A bra that has a plastic barrel closure or zipper in the front instead of the typical hook-and-eye closure in the back.

Full-Coverage Bra: A bra with cups that extend well above the nipple. This is the best bra style for larger breasts because it provides more coverage and support.

Graduated Padding: A bra-padding technique in which more padding is used near the bottom of the cup and then gradually lightened towards the top, providing a more natural looking push-up. In traditional padded bras, the cup is padded evenly all over.

Hidden Underwire Bra: A bra that has no seam separating the cups from the underwire, concealing the underwire from view and often offering greater comfort to the wearer.

Inner Sling: A soft strip of fabric inside a bra that follows the bottom curve of the cup, similar to an underwire, to provide added support.

Kleenex: A type of padding once used by teenage girls to "stuff their bras." With all the padding options out there today (see *Cookie, Cutlet,* and *Push-Up Bra*), Kleenex is rarely needed anymore—at least for this purpose!

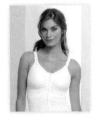

Lace: An ornamental fabric made of net-like threads sewn by hand or machine. It is often used in bras and other lingerie to create a sexy appearance.

Lycra: A stretch fiber, or spandex, that is a registered trademark of Invista, formerly DuPont. It is the most recognized and popular brand of spandex throughout the world, and many designers and clothing manufacturers use it in their products. Lycra is used in fabric blends alongside cotton, silk, and synthetic fibers, and is popular in bras and swimwear. It allows garments to be more lightweight, comfortable, and breathable. It is also quick-drying and resistant to bacteria, ultraviolet (UV) rays, and chlorine.

Mastectomy Bra: A bra that is specially designed for women who have had one or more breasts removed in surgery, called a mastectomy. It has special pockets to hold a prosthesis breast, or "mastectomy form," in place.

Maternity Bra: A bra that is specially designed for women who are pregnant. It offers wider straps to increase support and reduce bounce, as well as more comfortable material to prevent breast tissue irritation, since pregnant women often have swelling and tenderness in the breasts. Oftentimes, maternity and nursing bras are one and the same, so the bra will also include clasps on the front of each strap to allow the cup to be

37

pulled down. This allows you to breastfeed without having taking off your entire bra.

Microfiber: A fabric often used in bras, especially t-shirt bras. According to atlastbras.com, microfiber is "made from polyester and polyamide that's finer than the finest silk thread. [Its threads] are particularly soft, pliable and pleasant on the skin, offering maximum comfort."

Minimizer: A bra designed for larger-breasted women who wish to create the illusion of smaller breasts. According to intimateguide.com, this bra "reduces the projection of the wearer's breasts by holding the breast tissue snugly and redistributing breast flesh more towards the underarm and the center front."

Molded Cup: A bra cup that is created by a heat and pressure process that molds fabric into shape. Also known as seamless cups (because the process results in no visible fabric seams), molded cups are often found

38

in contour bras and in t-shirt bras, and are nearly invisible under clothes.

N

Nursing Bra: A bra that is specially designed for women who are nursing. Like a maternity bra, it offers extra support, but it also has cup openings to allow for breastfeeding without removing the entire bra.

O

Oprah Winfrey: Television's longtime talk show queen, credited with putting bras back in the spotlight when she declared America needed a "bra intervention" in 2005.

P

Pasties: A decorative covering that is meant to conceal just the nipple while leaving the rest of the breast bare. It is usually applied with a special glue or tape.

Plunge Bra: A bra with a center that dips low between the breasts in front so that only cleavage is revealed under low-cut garments.

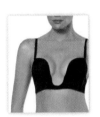 Fashion Forms makes a "U"-cut version with a lower-than-normal band that allows the center to dip several inches below the middle of the breasts.

Push-Up Bra: A bra with padded cups that is designed to press the breasts upward and create a fuller appearance.

Q is the quest for the perfect bra. You are one step closer, simply by reading this book!

Racerback Bra: A bra with straps that form a Y-shape in the back. It's useful for concealing straps under

THE ABCs OF BRAS FAST FACT

There are at least 374 words in the English language that start with "bra." These include brace, brag, brainstorm, brave, and of course, brassiere!

sleeveless clothing, since the straps aren't as wide-set in the front as a normal bra's.

Rayon: A synthetic silk-like fabric that is used in bras and many articles of clothing because of its low cost and high versatility.

 Satin: A smooth fabric of silk or rayon that is often used in bras. It has a glossy face and a dull back.

Silicone: A clear compound used in gel pads that are placed into bra cups to increase bust size, in some breast implants, and on

39

the inside of the band on strapless bras to prevent slippage by "gripping" the skin. It is composed of both organic and inorganic polymers, and is created through a specific chemical formula.

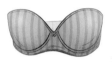

Strapless Bra: An underwire bra with no straps that is often worn with special occasion attire or other complicated tops where bra straps would be visible. This bra *sounds* simple (i.e., a bra without straps), but it can be difficult to find one that fits properly and doesn't slide down the body when worn.

40

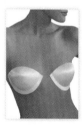

Support Adhesive: A lightweight foam bra "cup" that is coated with adhesive so it can stick to the skin, providing bra-like support without the bulk of a full bra.

T-Shirt Bra: A bra with molded cups that is often smooth and seamless so it appears "invisible" under t-shirts or other thin tops.

Underwire: A piece of metal that is sewn into the bra under the cup to lift and shape the bust. It is used as an additional means of supporting the breasts.

Viscose: A soft rayon fabric that is very similar to cotton or silk. It is made from purified cellulose, which usually comes from specially processed wood pulp.

X-Back Bra: A bra with straps that crisscross in the back to form an X-shape. Much like the racerback or Y-back bra, it allows the wearer to avoid showing her straps in tops that have narrow shoulders and backs (and prevents her straps from slipping off her shoulders).

Zip-Front Bra: A bra that closes with a zipper in the front. Zip-fronts usually only appear on sports bras.

THE PROCESS

Understanding how new bra designs come to fruition can also help you understand how and why bras work the way they do. Every new design begins with a concept—like a bra with an extra-deep plunge—which is conceived and crafted by a bra designer. After a concept is conceived, a technical design is sketched and a pattern is created. From that pattern, a prototype or "working model" is crafted by machines or by hand, or a combination of both, depending on what the design entails. The methods of making a prototype vary from company to company. Often a pair of cups is formed by "hot pressing" foam into the proper shape. Then the other parts, such as the band and straps, are sewed on. This prototype often goes through many incarnations to get the details just right and to make sure every part is not just fashionable, but functional.

Once the prototype is refined, a live "fit model" is brought in. The model tries the prototype on and describes what the bra feels like to wear: where it's comfortable, where the fit feels off. The design is then adjusted if necessary.

After that, the designers, manufacturers, and marketing team collaborate to ensure they have a sellable product that will appeal to as many women as possible. They all want the new bra to be "the next big thing" and, obviously, make a profit.

FIT MODELS

The standard fit model for bras is a size 34B. To determine the dimensions for all the other sizes, "They scale up or down from that," says Marla Greene, a New York–based former bra buyer. "For large size/full figure bras, they actually use either a 36C or 38C model. The full figure styles cannot be scaled up from a 34B since it is an entirely different fit, frame, and cup capacity. Each vendor uses different frames and cup capacities and they all vary." Since fit models are only human, it's safe to say that if the model's size is a little "off" (for example, she's not an exact "B"), then the brand's sizes could be a little off, too. Many experts believe this is part of the reason fit varies from brand to brand and even between styles within each brand.

FABRIC AND MATERIALS

While design is important, improvements in fabrics and materials are just as essential. The first bras were made out of a cotton-based material; then came nylons and satin. Today, there are many more fabric options to choose from, offering benefits from increased durability to better stretch. There are even new fabrics that are better for the environment!

WHY WE LOVE LYCRA

In 1959 Lycra, a stretchy synthetic spandex fiber known for its exceptional elasticity, hit the market, and has since proved to be perhaps the most useful fabric ever invented. Not only has Lycra improved comfort and flexibility, it's also given wearers increased durability—something consumers crave, according to a survey by Lycra commissioned in the UK. It showed that 32 percent of bra-buyers want an "indestructible" bra that can be machine-washed without fading or fraying. Invista, the company that makes Lycra, responded with the introduction of Lycra Black, an elastane fiber that prevents the color from fading in the wash thanks to its spun-dyed technology. It also reduces the "shiny" uneven effect that can occur when dark Lycra is stretched.

Unfortunately, while these Lycra bras can withstand more wear and tear than their predecessors and still retain their shape (Lycra can be stretched up to four to seven times its original length and still spring back once released), they still won't stand the test of time when you're talking about repeated washings and wearing. They aren't quite "indestructible" yet!

Lycra has also contributed to recent innovations in nursing bras. Their cups are now frequently made of a stretchy cotton/Lycra blend to allow for the many changes breastfeeding women experience as their breasts engorge and deplete.

A MORE PLEASANT PADDING

Bra padding used to be made of cloth, until bra manufacturers realized gel and air pockets could provide more comfortable, natural-looking bulk. But the latest padding innovation has been the use of foam, which achieves the same effect without weighing down the bra (or the wearer!).

Foam has also changed the bra industry in other ways. Many bra cups today are lined with thin stretch foam, made of non-allergenic material, rather than fabric. Foam is what allows molded cup bras to retain their shape at all times while maintaining a smooth appearance under tops, and is also thinner than fiberfill lining, so it prevents nipple show-through without adding extra bulk.

WHEN THE MERCURY'S RISING

A fifth of the women in that Lycra survey said they wanted their bras to anticipate their needs by heating up or cooling down as external temperatures changed. While nothing quite like this has appeared in the marketplace yet, moisture-wicking fabrics, traditionally reserved for exercise apparel, are now making a splash in the everyday bra market because they keep wearers cool and dry. So-called "intelligent fabrics" like Coolmax, Double Dry, PlayDry, and 02Cool (nearly every company has their own patented moisture-wicking fabric) allow these bras to work with the temperature of your body. Most work by pulling perspiration from your skin and then drawing the moisture to the outside of the fabric, where it runs off or evaporates. Microfiber fabrics, usually made of either a nylon or polyester blend, can have a similar "cooling effect" because the fabrics breathe well—they absorb and release perspiration quickly.

OTHER MATERIAL INNOVATIONS

Innovations are being made in materials for other parts of the bra, too, especially the underwire. In most bras, the metal underwire (made from heavy gauge wire or sheet metal) are wrapped in gel or plastic. While this helps cushion the wearer, underwire can still not only break, but also poke through the fabric of the bra and cause pain. So bra-makers have been on a quest to find alternate materials.

Molded plastic is now being used in place of metal entirely in many bras because of its pliability. In 2000 London-based product design and research company SeymourPowell used automobile machinery to gather data on breast shape and form and develop a molded-plastic piece to replace traditional underwire. The firm identified an "ouch zone" under the arm where underwires frequently dig into bra wearers, and developed "plastic wings" to alleviate this problem. The design of the underwire was modeled after a chicken's two-piece breast bone and replaced twenty-four separate pieces found in traditional underwire bras. While their design made headlines when it was put on the market as the Bioform bra by lingerie retailer Charnos, it was ultimately too expensive to make and in the end fell flat with buyers.

However, the concept of using plastic in place of metal stuck. Instead of rigid pieces of metal with the potential to poke out and cause pain, today's plastic and metal wire-wrapped-plastic underwire is flexible, encased in foam, and stays in place, hidden within the molded piece in a way that reduces the risk of the wire popping out. This new technique is referred to as a "hidden underwire." Hidden underwire also creates a sleeker silhouette and a more comfortable bra altogether. Warner's Elements of Bliss underwire bra features a soft underwire that's wrapped in three layers of fabric for increased comfort.

Straps have also been a recent site of innovation. Some bras now come with straps lined in a material such as silicone that grips the wearer's skin to keep straps from slipping. Another innovation: new gel-strap

45

bras have straps that are infused with
silicone gel to disperse pressure more evenly,
relieving shoulder strain and preventing
straps from digging in.

Now that you've learned the basics, you're ready to move on to the most important aspect
of the bra: fit! Read on for the *dos* and *don'ts* of bra fit, and how to make sure you're
wearing the right size.

three

Like a Glove

(for Boobs)

Finding the Perfect Fit

As we know, not all busts are created equal. That's why, when it comes to bras, there are several different cup sizes and band measurements for a woman to choose from, to ensure her bra is a perfect fit. But what really constitutes a "perfect" fit, and does such perfection exist? Most experts will tell you that it's tough to attain "perfection" when it comes to bras, short of spending hundreds of dollars to have one custom-made for your body. But what you can do is follow some simple rules to at least find one that fits you well.

Chances are the bra you are wearing now *doesn't*. Statistics show (and Oprah said it, too) that 85 percent of us are wearing the wrong bra size altogether! But how could that be? "I have been a 34C for years!" you say. This common denial could be costing you the comfort and support you deserve. I was smug when I met with Frederika Zappe, the nationally renowned bra fit expert for Eveden, when I first began the journey of writing this book. I was convinced she wasn't going to tell *me* anything new. But boy was I ever wrong! Wrong cup size, wrong band measurement—you guessed it—wrong bra! Once she put me in the right size, I immediately looked thinner and more proportioned, and even my posture improved. A co-worker the next day even asked me if I had lost weight!

Since then, I've worked with hundreds of women at personal appearances and events, and I can attest that rarely do I meet one who is in the perfectly right style and/or size! I love seeing the looks of shock on their faces once they're wearing the bra that's right for them, and always encourage them to follow up with me to see how they are faring in their "new" sizes.

The information and tips in this chapter will help you understand how your bra is supposed to fit and why it's so important to get it right. And in the end, even if you haven't yet achieved "perfection," at least you'll be standing a little taller.

WHY DO WE GET IT WRONG?

· ·

Finding the right bra is like finding a good man. Many women I know are consistently choosing Mr. Wrong. And after years in a bad relationship, they go right out and find another man who doesn't call when he says he will, shows clear disregard for their feelings, and ultimately breaks their hearts. While our bras aren't likely to break our hearts, they can let us down, failing us when we need them the most. And although they won't forget our anniversary, they certainly won't last us till the next one (it's recommended we replace our bras every six months to a year).

I can't explain why women continue to choose the wrong men (I'll leave that one to Siggy Flicker), but I can offer up two main explanations as to why we consistently choose the wrong bra.

The first has to do with size. Figuring out your correct size is tough, and most of us don't know what a properly sized bra really looks like.

The second has to do with budget. Bras may be skimpy, but they're nothing to skimp on. Most women feel that a "good" bra is too much of an investment of their hard-earned cash. But don't let your pocketbook affect your judgment. You certainly don't need to spend $100 on a great bra—just $40-$50 is usually fine! But you need to look at the money you spend on a new bra the same the way you do, say, the money you spend tuning up your car. You wouldn't drive around in a car that's low on oil, would you? It stresses the car's system and can cost even more cash in the end! Plus, avoiding the daily discomfort of an ill-fitting bra is worth the money all on its own. So just take some time once a year or so, go get a fitting, and invest in some new bras. You'll be much better off!

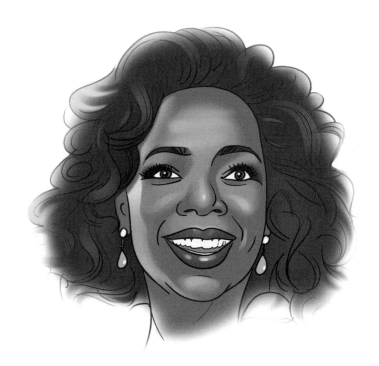

"America, you are wearing the wrong bra!"
—Oprah Winfrey

How You Can Tell You Are

If 85 percent of us are wearing the wrong one, chances are most of us don't even know it. The first rule of thumb? If your bra causes you pain in any way, it doesn't fit properly.

Here are some other basic warning signs that you are wearing an ill-fitting bra (plus solutions for each):

FROM THE BACK

The Problem: The shoulder straps fall down or dig in.
The Solution: The straps may simply need to be adjusted. Or in the case of dig-in, you may need a larger band or cup size.

The Problem: The band either rides up or slides down in the back, instead of remaining somewhat "level" all the way around your body, or squeezes your flesh in a way that causes pain or leaves marks.
The Solution: You likely need a different band size. If the bra band slides downward, you need a smaller size; if it rides up or causes bulging, you may need to go larger.

52

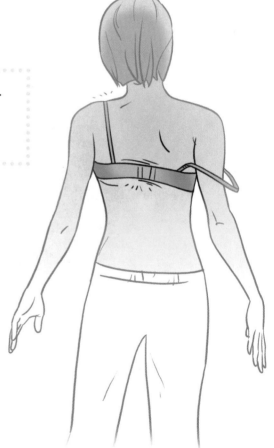

Wearing the Wrong One

FROM THE FRONT

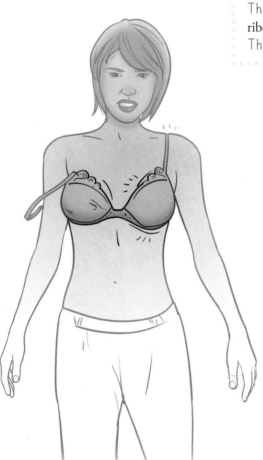

The Problem: The underwire isn't flush against your ribcage or is cutting into the underside of your breasts.
The Solution: You need a larger cup size.

The Problem: The bridge of the bra doesn't lie flat against your body.
The Solution: You need a larger cup size.

The Problem: Your nipples pop out of the cups, or your breast tissue billows out of the top, creating a "double boob" effect.
The Solution: You need either a larger cup size or a fuller-coverage cup.

The Problem: The cups are baggy, gaping, or wrinkly.
The Solution: You need a smaller cup size. However, minor gaping at the top of cups can sometimes be eliminated by tightening your straps, so be sure to try that first!

53

HOW TO FIND THE RIGHT ONE

Your first step in finding the right bra is getting "sized up." Visit a bra or lingerie store that has bra fitters on hand, and let them work their magic (leave your modesty at home). Many women have never been fitted at all, while others haven't been fitted in a long time. It's important to remember that due to changes in our bodies (which will be discussed in detail in Chapters 5 and 6), you need to get re-fitted every six months to a year!

Most malls contain a Victoria's Secret, which specially trains employees on how to fit bras in its very own "bra room." Department stores like Neiman Marcus,

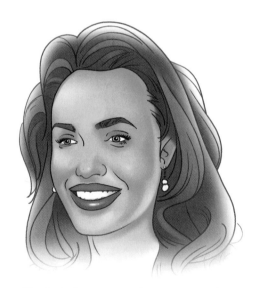

"I didn't even know my bra size until I made a movie."
—Angelina Jolie

Macy's, and Bloomingdale's also often have lingerie departments (JCPenney recently expanded theirs!) with employees who are equipped to take your measurements (in the case of Bloomingdale's, they are actually "certified"). And it's free! Another option is to visit a local seamstress and have her measure you. But for starters, you can get a rough approximation of your size by measuring yourself.

The most important thing is to get educated *before* you walk into the store, so that the salesperson is merely there to assist you, as opposed to relying on the store's salesperson completely (in some cases, you will know more than they do). The end result will be the best possible bra for you!

HOW BRA SIZES WORK

Your bra size contains two important parts:

▶ An even number that represents the circumference of your ribcage below your breasts and describes your band size

▶ A letter that describes your cup size

While this sounds simple, it isn't. There are many misconceptions about what these numbers mean.

LIKE A GLOVE FIT TIP

What about strapless? A great-fitting strapless bra can be tricky to find. But it's easy to tell when it's wrong—it's either sliding down your body and off your breasts completely, or it's cutting your breasts horizontally, giving you the dreaded "four-boobs." Look for one that has silicone around the entire inside of the band and the tops of the cups for extra staying power. And don't forget to skip lotions and oils the day you plan to wear it!

55

For starters, band size doesn't necessarily equal the number of inches your ribcage measures around. Your band size is estimated *based* on the width of your ribcage, but it isn't an exact science. You often have to add one or two inches to

LIKE A GLOVE FIT TIP

The secret to strapless? Going down a band size in a strapless bra for better support. If you are a 34B, for example, try purchasing a 32B. Just make sure it's still comfortable and not cutting off your circulation!

get your correct band size, depending on manufacturer and style. A 34 in one bra may feel just right while a 34 in another may be too tight. (I'll explain in greater detail in the sizing section that follows.)

Also adding to the confusion: If you stretch a bra out in its entirety and measure the band, that measurement typically won't match up to the band size. So, for example, the bra may be a 34 band, but stretched out, its band won't actually measure 34 inches.

Figuring out your cup size isn't easy either. It's calculated *in relation to* your band size. The size of an A-cup—the volume an A-cup holds—changes depending on the band size. An A-cup on a 32 band is not the same as an A-cup on a 34 band, and so on.

Let's say you are in your favorite lingerie store and you spot a bra you absolutely *have* to have. However, you are a 34C and they don't have your size. What to do? Because of the way bra sizing works, you may be able to try "sister sizing." Because bra sizes are based on volume, you can go down a band size and up a cup size and still achieve a similar fit. If your band size is small enough that many bra makers don't carry it, you can also try going up a band size and down a cup size, although that's not typically recommended—you always want a snug band to get the best possible fit and to allow for stretch and give as you wear it. Just because a B is thought to be smaller than a C doesn't mean it actually is. A B is just smaller than a C in the same band size. Why? The snugger band size decreases the width and depth of the cup, which means the 34C, while smaller than the 36C, actually holds the same *volume* of breast tissue as the 36B. This trick can be particularly useful for larger cup sizes. For

BUYING BRAS OVERSEAS

While sizes vary by manufacturer, they also vary by country. With the internet making international shopping easy, and more U.S. stores importing international brands, you may find that you want to buy a European- or Australian-made bra. Check the charts below for your international size conversion.

BRAS – BAND SIZES

USA	UK	Euro	French	Italian	Australian
28	28				
30	30				
32	32	70	85	1	10
34	34	75	90	2	12
36	36	80	95	3	14
38	38	85	100	4	16
40	40	90	105	5	18
42	42				
44	44				
46	46				
48	48				
50	50				
52	52				
54	54				
56	56				

BRAS – CUP SIZES

USA	UK	Euro	French	Italian	Australian
AA	AA	AA	AA		
A	A	A	A	A	A
B	B	B	B	B or None	B
C	C	C	C	C	C
D	D	D	D	D	D
DD/E	DD	E	E	DD	DD
DDD/F	E	F	F	E	E
G	FF			F	F
H	FF				FF
I	G				G
J	GG				GG
K	H				HH
L	HH				
M	J				J
N	JJ				JJ
	K				

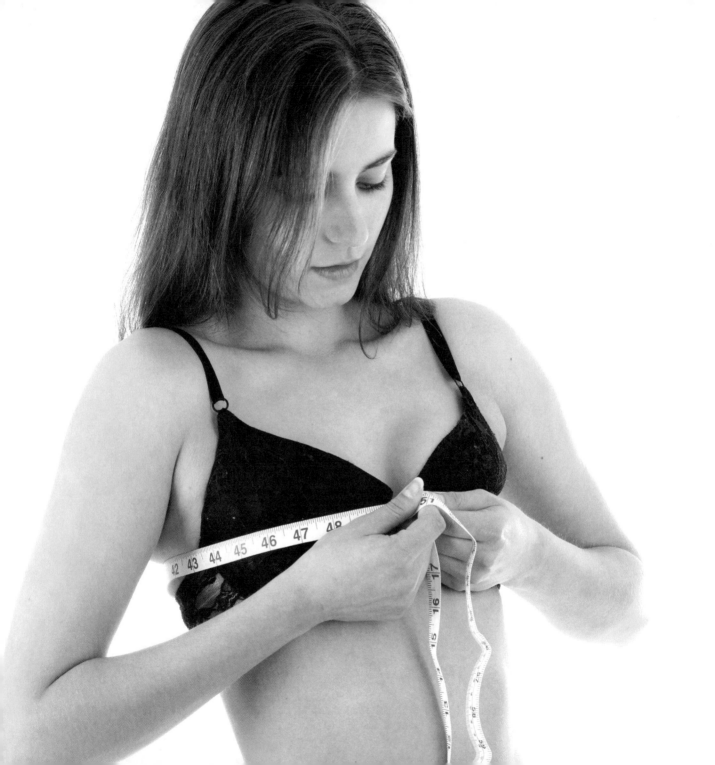

example, after my first pregnancy, I was wearing a 34G, which can be a tough size to find. When I found a bra style I really liked and it didn't come in a G cup, I opted to try the 36F instead. It worked perfectly!

The best way to really understand this is to go into a store and compare bra cups on different size bands. If you compare a 38A to a 34A, the 38A's cup will be obviously bigger. But if you compare a 38A and 34D, the cups will be much closer in size. This doesn't mean that these two sizes are interchangeable, however; you still need to wear the correct band size for proper support.

Thankfully, there is no measurement needed for the shoulder straps, as they are adjustable on every bra. At least one part of this is easy!

YOUR BRA SIZE

To find the bra size you should be wearing, you'll need a tape measure (the kind you use in sewing, not the kind that comes in the tool box) to obtain the measurements we'll use to determine your band and cup sizes. You can find one at most drugstores for a couple of dollars.

Step 1: Band Size

First, wrap the tape measure around your ribcage just below your bust (be sure to exhale first) and take the measurement. Since bra band sizes are even numbers, round up to the nearest. For example, if you measure at an odd 31 inches, round up to 32.

Now comes the complicated part. The most common way of fitting advises you to add 4 inches to this number, but this method doesn't always work. Some theorize that this "old standby" fitting rule was devised back when bras were made with less stretch, before more pliable fabrics and materials were invented, and as a result, women who use this method often end up in bras with band sizes that are too big to offer them the proper support. What works better for many women is to add only two inches to their rounded-up ribcage measurement. So if you measure at 30 inches, you are likely a 32 band size.

Some fitting methods actually combine these two, advising that if your ribcage measurement is a 32 or below, then add 4 inches, and if it's a 34 or above, add only 2. (Mostly, however, that's just because bra designers don't make a whole lot of sizes. If

59

DIFFERENCE BUST MEASUREMENT MINUS BAND SIZE	U.S. CUP SIZE
Less than 1"	AA
1"	A
2"	B
3"	C
4"	D
5"	DD/E
6"	DDD/F
7"	G
7.5"	GG
8"	G, H
9"	H, I
10"	H, I, J
11"	HH
11.5" – 13"	I
13" – 15.5"	J
15.5" – 17"	K, JJ

In sizes above DD, the same cup size is often referred to by several different letters, as shown above. So if you wear a DDD in one brand, you may wear an F in another.

you're a 30F, for example, you may just have a tough time finding viable options in your size; going up to a 34 rather than a 32 band increases your buying options. Just don't forget to adjust the cup size accordingly!) Still other fitters will advise you not to add any additional inches at all—which does work for some women. For example, I measure exactly at a 34, and that is the band size I wear.

Why all the discrepancy? Bra bands are often not "true to size"—for example, if you stretch out a 32-inch band bra and measure it, it won't actually be 32 inches long.

So what should you do? Pick whatever method you feel fits you best for now, but treat the size you get as a starting point only. Be prepared to go up or down in band size (and to recalculate your cup size accordingly), depending on the vendor and the style, to find that perfect fit. Use your size as a guideline and be sure to try on bras before you buy.

Step 2: Cup Size

Next, wrap the tape measure around the fullest part of your bust. Then subtract your band size from this number, and use the difference in inches to calculate your cup size using the chart in the left column. For example, if your bust measurement is an inch larger than your band size, your cup size will most likely be an A; if your bust measurement is two inches larger than your band size, your cup size will most likely be a B; and so on.

One question I get asked a lot: Can you measure your cup size while wearing a bra and shirt? I say yes. It helps you find your cup size while boobs are boosted and at their perkiest.

Step 3: Try and Buy

Finally, try out your new size. Go to the store and grab various bras in the size you have measured for yourself. If you're above a DD, chances are you will have to shop online, as many stores don't carry above this size, although this is changing as time goes on. Make sure to pick a store with a great return policy so you can still try your new size out before committing to buy.

So many women make the mistake of approaching bra shopping as if they're going grocery shopping. They go to the store, pluck something they like from the shelf, and buy it, expecting it to fit like a glove, only to be disappointed when they return home and find it doesn't. Think about it—would you

LIKE A GLOVE FIT TIP

If you opt to order online, as many people do, be sure that the store has a good return policy and that you are familiar with it before you order. (One website I frequent requires that tags still be attached when you return, and I have this habit of ripping them off immediately, making them nonreturnable.)

buy a pair of shoes without trying them on? And those are just for your feet!

In bras, as in any article of clothing, so-called "standard" sizes can vary. For example, you're used to wearing a certain size, such as a size 10. But often, you'll go to the store to try on a dress or a pair of pants and end up going home with a size 12. We're not used to thinking that way when it comes to bras, but we should be.

FITTING UNEVEN BREASTS

What do you do if one of your breasts is larger (or smaller) than the other? This is a very common problem for many women; on average, women have one breast that's about half a cup size bigger than the other. But just because it's common doesn't mean it's always easy to fix. Surgery is one available option, but a more short-term solution is to fit your bra cup to the larger breast and then add some light padding or a silicone bra insert known as a cutlet to the cup on the smaller breast. Pre-surgery, I used to buy bras with removable pads and simply remove the pad on the side that was larger. Also, be sure to tighten the strap a little more on the side with the larger breast—you want to make sure it's as supported as possible.

LIKE A GLOVE FIT TIP

If you find a bra you really like but it's a bit off in the fit, you can usually get it "customized" for just a few dollars. Some stores have a seamstress on hand who will tailor your purchases for a truly perfect fit, or you can always take a trip to the neighborhood tailor. (Believe me, there is nothing to be embarrassed about. Most likely, they have altered bras before.)

"You can be three different sizes in a bra," says Alicia Vargo, founder of lingerie company Pampered Passions. "Just like a pair of blue jeans or a favorite shirt, you can be many different sizes depending on who makes the bra and how their sizing system works. We have all been trained that size comes first and matters most, when in essence it's the fit of a brand that matters first and foremost." Bras fit differently depending on the manufacturer, and both band and cup sizes can be a bit off. If you got fitted at Victoria's Secret, you may require a different size altogether when you're at a department store trying on their brands.

Moral of the story? Try on each and every bra you want to buy *before* you leave the store. I suggest finding the style and size that you feel most comfortable in and stocking up. But it's important to note that even if you find a brand you like, different styles *within* that brand may vary, too—so you still need to try on any bra you're planning to buy. Only go bra shopping when you have at least an hour to spare and try, try, try! I know, you're busy, but aren't your "girls" important?

One final bra-shopping tip: Wear or bring along a t-shirt or tank top to try on over the bra—it'll be easy to spot any poor-fit red flags like bulges, etc., through the thin fabric.

63

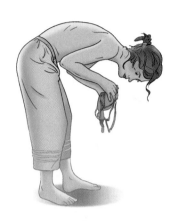

Step 1

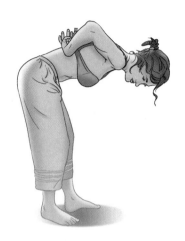

Step 2

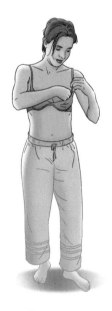

Step 3

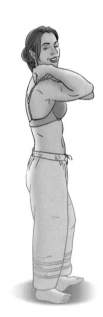

Step 4

HOW TO
PUT YOUR BRA ON

It's also important to know how to properly *put on* your bra. Even if you have the right size, a bra may not fit properly because your breasts are not sitting correctly in the cups and the straps aren't adjusted the way they should be. So what's the proper way to put on a bra? It can be done in four simple steps:

Step 1: Bend over until you are almost touching your toes, so that all of your breast tissue falls forward.

Step 2: While still bent over, slip the straps over your shoulders, and then hook the band on the tightest row that is comfortable (you should still be able to fit one or two fingers between the band and your body).

Step 3: Put your hand underneath each breast and "scoop" it toward the middle and into the bra's cup. This ensures your breasts are properly settled into the cups. (This step is so important! You will notice the difference immediately, I promise.)

Step 4: Stand up and adjust the straps!

Remember that you'll likely have to adjust the shoulder straps every time you put the bra on, since wearing or washing can affect your straps' "setting."

How You Can Tell That It Fits

Here's what a proper-fitting bra looks like:

FROM THE FRONT

Underwire lies flat against the ribcage, and rests on bone (not breast tissue) on both sides

Breast tissue is perfectly settled into the cups so that there is no bulging or gaping

Bridge lies flat between the breasts

FROM THE BACK

Back of band is straight across and not riding up or squeezing flesh

Straps lay perfectly in place without digging in

66

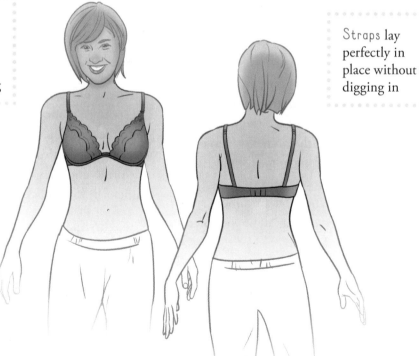

LIKE A GLOVE FIT TIP:
THE PERFECT BRA IN UNDER 3 MINUTES!

Finding the right bra online can be tough, especially given the importance of trying on. But websites like ThirdLove and True&Co—and even apps for your smart phone!—aim to make the process a little easier. Just go to ThirdLove. com and click on the "My Fit" tab or go to TrueandCo.com and click on the "Get Fitted" tab. Answer a short series of very specific questions related to breast shape, bra fit, feel, and size, and these sites will recommend the "perfect" bras for you that you can order right then and there. It's sort of like a Match.com for bras! ThirdLove.com even factors bra *shape* into the sizing equation, as well as offering bras in half-cup sizes for those who are in between sizes.

67

You can also determine if your bra is fitting properly by checking where your breasts are sitting in relation to the rest of your upper body. If they are being supported correctly, the fullest part of your breasts should be positioned halfway between your shoulder and your elbow.

Comfort is Key. Make sure it feels comfortable when you sit down and when you move your arms up, over your head, and sideways.

Looks Are Important, Too! Always try bras on while wearing a thin t-shirt—it's the best way to see what a bra is doing (or not

LIKE A GLOVE FIT TIP

Most bra fitters recommend you fit your bra so that it hooks comfortably on the middle hook, allowing you to extend to an outside hook if you gain a little weight, and an inside hook if you lose some or the band stretches.

68

doing) for you. Every bit of lace, boning, underwire, and seam can make a difference in the way you look in your bra, and under the barest t-shirt each one will show clearly. (This is also a good way to check for back and side "bulges" and other maladies.)

The Perfect Fit. Your breasts should feel like they are "sitting" upright in the cups. You should not feel any underwire pinching and your bra should feel comfortable and supportive.

Now that you've mastered your everyday bra's fit, it's time to delve into a special case: the sports bra.

SPORTS SUPPORT

Sports bras have been around for thirty years yet are still a mystery to most women. But proper fit and support is just as important in a sports bra as in the everyday model—maybe more! Researchers say an unsupported breast can move up and down about six centimeters when we're working out. Not a good thing for the girls.

Whether you're a jogger, a dancer, a kickboxer, or a yoga enthusiast, you need a well-fitting sports bra that keeps your breasts firmly in place when you move—even if you're a small-breasted woman! Actress Katie Holmes raised eyebrows when she appeared to be braless while running the New York City marathon. It's always a good idea to support any and all breast tissue with a proper-fitting sports bra, even if you feel like you don't need it.

Sports bras generally come in two basic designs: encapsulation and compression.

Sound scientific? Well, they are. These "models" have been developed as a result of research like the study from Chapter 2, and each is designed to minimize movement of the breasts in a different way. When you wear the compression style, the most common type of sports bra, your breasts are pressed together, flat against your chest, to reduce motion. This option best suits

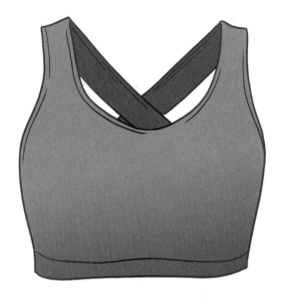

Compression

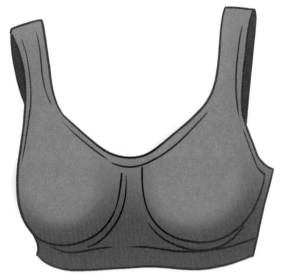

Encapsulation

70

smaller-breasted women (up to a D-cup) as compression sports bras can often be too "constraining," and less effective, for larger-breasted women. Compression-style bras come sized small, medium, or large. Usually, a small correlates to a 32B/C, a medium to a 34B/C, and a large to a 36B/C. If you are an A, try on the small. If you are a D or larger, try a large or extra-large. In some cases, the extra-large won't be big enough, so you'll want to look for a sports bra that comes

in your exact band and cup size— like an encapsulation-style sports bra.

Encapsulation sports bras are sized like regular bras, by both band and cup size. According to a 2006 article by Thomas Affatato on www.infinitehealthresources. com, "encapsulation models are constructed with two cups (just like typical bras), under the theory that two small masses are easier to control than one large one." Experts say this is the better option for women whose breasts are larger than a D-cup, as this type offers more support by compressing each breast separately.

If you're in the store, you can usually tell which style is which. Compression bras are usually one piece and designed to be pulled on over your head, whereas encapsulation bras have actual "cups" and often an underwire as well. Keep in mind that, no matter which style you choose, sports bras are meant to feel snugger than your normal bra, but they shouldn't be so tight that they irritate your skin.

Sports bras are infamous for creating a uniboob appearance (especially the compression models) but many on the market today are much more flattering. Plus, many sports bras are even chic enough to wear by themselves! You'll stay cooler in them that way, too. I have taken a liking to styles that zip up in the front—you can adjust your breast tissue after you zip it up and create great cleavage, sans uniboob effect. But whichever style you choose, it's important to shop around and get the best fit you can.

Here are some tips for finding a great-fitting sports bra:

> ## LIKE A GLOVE FIT TIP
> Your sports bra's tag can be a wealth of information. In addition to listing size and material, sometimes it even tells you what activities the bra is designed for.

71

▶ Make sure the elastic band on the bottom fits snugly around your ribcage, but not so snugly that you can't breathe.

▶ Jump up and down a few times in the dressing room. You may look a little crazy, but you'll accurately determine if the bra gives you the amount of support needed for physical activity! Obviously, the less "bounce," the better. The sports bra, more than any other bra, is all about limiting range of motion.

▶ Look for wider shoulder straps for increased support.

LIKE A GLOVE FAST FACT

A Harris survey commissioned by Playtex asked more than 1,000 women what they like in a bra. Sixty-seven percent said they prefer wearing a bra over going braless. Eighty-five percent said they want a "shape-enhancing bra that feels like nothing at all." On the issue of underwire, ladies were split. Forty-nine percent said they prefer underwire while 49 percent said they prefer to do without.

72

► Note that those with built-in "shock absorbers" are designed to minimize bounce.

The fabric you choose also has an impact on the comfort and effectiveness of the sports bra—most are designed to wick moisture away from the body, but you can choose one that also goes a step further by preventing chafing and all-around discomfort. Check the tag before you buy so you know what your sports bra is made of.

According to www.olympiasports.net, there are several different fabrics to choose from. Here is a breakdown of the options, with the most common first:

Polyester/Cotton: This classic blend provides gentle softness and powerful moisture management for all your workouts.

Cotton/Lycra: This combination of soft, moisture-managing cotton and shape-retaining Lycra creates a very comfortable fabric with just the right amount of stretch and support.

CoolMax polyester/Lycra: This high-performance fabric blend delivers you all the moisture-wicking benefits of

MAKING AN IMPACT

Different activities have different impacts on our bodies (and our breasts), so many sports bras are designed with that in mind. Here is a guideline so you know what type of sports bra to look for, depending on the activity:

LOW IMPACT

Walking

Yoga

Bicycling or spinning

Weight training

Low-impact aerobics

MEDIUM IMPACT

Skiing

Skating

Tennis

Golf

HIGH IMPACT

Aerobics

Running

Mountain biking

Softball

Soccer

Basketball

Horseback riding

Kickboxing/boxing

CoolMax plus the comfort, stretch, and shape retention of Lycra.

Polyester/Cotton/Lycra: This three-fiber blend offers polyester and cotton for softness and moisture management while Lycra provides optimal fit and support.

Supplex nylon/Lycra: This blend offers soft, luxurious feel and incredible fit, support, and shape retention.

Because of wear and tear, sports bras should also be replaced at least every year, depending on how much use they get. How do you know if it's time for a new one? Tell-tale signs are if the elastic is stretched out and no longer flush against your ribcage or if you notice increased breast motion or pilling on the fabric.

BRA FIT CHEAT SHEET

Just to recap, here are the three most important points to remember when it comes to bra fit:

▶ See a Pro. Seeing a professional for measurements will help ensure you figure out the correct size. A professional can also help you weave your way through the maze of brassieres that promise to lift, separate, and even mimic a boob job!

▶ Don't Get Stuck in a Size-Rut. You need to get re-fitted every six months to a year! Our breasts are constantly changing as we age and gain or lose weight, and especially after giving birth.

▶ Try Before You Buy. Bra sizes run differently depending on the brand, so even after you get fitted, you still need to try yours on to make sure it fits!

four

Going Undercover

Bras and Fashion

Fit isn't the only important factor when choosing the right bra. Much of our bra decisions revolve around fashion, as well. In fact, a survey by market research firm NPD Group showed that 66 percent of women choose the style and color of bra based on the clothes they'll be wearing.

Whether you're dressing for a special occasion or just for everyday life, you need to start with what's underneath! Bras are the first layer of your outfit and can have a huge effect on your overall appearance. "Creating the perfect foundation for your clothes is just as important as finding the perfect outfit," says Spanx founder Sara Blakely. Pick the right one—and your girls will look great no matter what you are wearing. (Disclaimer: We take no responsibility for that latex tube top.)

Just like you have different clothes for different occasions—like casual for the weekends, business for weekdays, and eveningwear for special events—you need different bras to meet different wardrobe needs. It would look really strange if you wore a push-up bra while working out, wouldn't it?

You should have a full arsenal of bras to fit your lifestyle, and in this chapter, we are going to present all the options. That way, you can decide for yourself what you need, based on the clothes in your closet.

BRA WARDROBE BASICS

According to Cyla Weiner, owner of Sylene, a lingerie store in Washington, D.C., "[every] woman should have at least seven different types of bras, one for each day of the week." Weiner uses a guideline that she calls the "s-factor": Each necessary bra begins with the letter "s." These seven staples serve as the foundation for your bra rotation:

One "Strapless" bra. The strapless bra is not just for eveningwear anymore. A strapless bra can be the one you use the most, especially if you get one that fits like a glove and is convertible— has removable straps—that allow you to wear it in a variety of ways, with a variety of outfits.

One "Spa" bra, for everyday comfort. T-shirt bras and contour bras fall into this category.

One "Specialty" bra, such as a plunge bra, for low-front tops and dresses.

One "Sports" bra.

Three "Sexy" bras, for evening, special occasions, and everyday work attire. This includes at least one demi-cup or balconette bra (for lower-cut tops) and at least one sheer or lacy (or whatever defines sexy to you!) full-coverage bra,

BRA FASHION FAST FACT

The bra wasn't always a wardrobe staple. Women didn't begin wearing them regularly until the early 1900s. At that time, bras were used to retain breasts, not enhance them, and women certainly weren't looking at them as a fashion item. By 1918, however, bras had become a fashion basic, and more than fifty different brands were available through department stores, in a plethora of styles.

for higher-cut tops. Note that demi cups are most flattering on small to medium busts, so if you have larger breasts you may want to look for some pretty full-coverage styles instead. Conversely, a smaller-busted woman may want to skip the full-coverage option and opt for a push-up instead!

Keep in mind: You'll want to adjust these recommendations for your own personal bra needs. If you are in casual wear the majority of the time, you'll want to stock up more on "Spa" bras, whereas a woman who spends 90 percent of her time in blouses and suits will want more of the dressier bras.

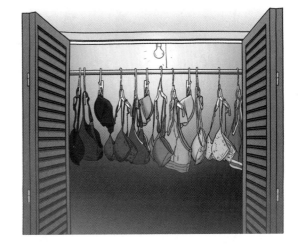

What to Wear *Under* There

Now that you know what bras you should have, you need to know what to wear them with. Knowing what goes under what can help you avert a major wardrobe malfunction.

Here is *The Bra Book*'s guide to what to wear under what (and if you need a little help on what each type of bra is, refer back to our bra alphabet in Chapter 2!):

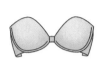

Backless strapless
bra

Balconette bra

Bandeau bra

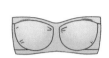

Bralette

Breast petals

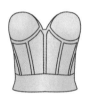

Bustier/Corset

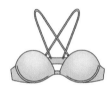

Convertible bra

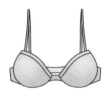

Demi-cup bra

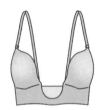

Plunge bra

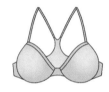

Racerback bra

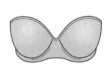

Strapless

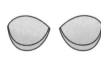

Support adhesives

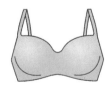

T-shirt bra

KEY

EVERYDAY

T-shirt or clingy top		A bra that's seamless, soft, and molded will stay invisible under thin fabric.
Sheer top		Unless you want the bra to show through, make sure it's nude-colored. Or if the top is black, wear a black bra!
Deep v-neck sweater		
Low-cut top	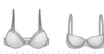	Which bra is best will depend on the cut of the top.
Backless or low-back top	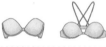	Look for a convertible where the band is also a strap that can wrap around the waist.
Boat neck top		
Off-the-shoulder top		
Tank top		
Sleeveless top		
Strapless top		

SPECIAL OCCASIONS

Gown or dress
with spaghetti straps

Halter dress or gown

You may need a convertible plunge bra in some cases, depending on how deep the neckline is.

One-shoulder
dress or gown

Wear one strap diagonally over the covered shoulder.

Strapless
dress or gown

Which bra is best will depend on the style of the dress.

Corset-style
dress or gown

Or go braless! This style usually has enough structure to support you on its own.

85

Dress or gown with
a plunging neckline

Backless
dress or gown

Dress or gown
that plunges in both
front and back

Dress or gown with a
strappy back and a sheer
or revealed midriff area

BRA FASHION FAST FACT

Corsets, the pain-inducing predecessors of the bra, were once used by women as a means of attaining a pushed up bosom and an unnaturally small waist. Now, corset styles are back in the fashion spotlight, gracing everything from evening gowns to blouses, and women are even investing in organ-crushing "waist cinchers" to actually shrink their waists over time. Sounds uncomfortable!

have to wear something and the bra you need just doesn't exist. Take this scenario, for example: Your friend asks you to be a bridesmaid in her wedding. She chooses the dress, and it's completely complicated. You give it a good eyeballing and know right off the bat it's not going to work with any of the bras you own—or any bra you've ever *seen*, for that matter. And it's not like you can just decide to *not* wear that dress. So what's the solution? Bra designer Tara Cavosie was in this exact same situation when she created the Backless Strapless Bra, which has become a staple for some women. But those of us who aren't quite as crafty can visit our local tailor. With a little snipping and some creative sewing, a seamstress can customize your bra exactly to your dress. Keep in mind, you should never sew your bra *into* your gown; as you move, *it* can move, and both bra and dress can end up looking pretty strange. However, seamstresses say sewn-in bra cups do work better for people whose cup sizes are smaller than a C, since things are less likely to shift out of place.

Although this list covers nearly every clothing style imaginable, sometimes you

COLOR-CODING

Technically a bra is underwear, which means it's not meant to be *seen* under your clothes. But the color bra you choose is still important. For one thing, your bra's color can greatly determine its visibility. You want your bra to go unnoticed . . . unless you're Rihanna, or just very daring (but hey, that's your prerogative).

Follow the chart on page 88 to determine what you can wear with each color bra. But first, two important rules regarding bra color:

In the Buff: You need at least two nude- or flesh-colored bras. (Why two? So you can rotate, or in case one is in the wash!) Contrary to popular belief, it's a nude bra that's the most versatile, not a white one. A white bra is fine for dark colors and thicker fabrics, but it usually shows under white tops. The nude bra, on the other hand, is inconspicuous under just about *everything*. And bras come in different shades of tan, beige, and brown, so you can find a perfect match regardless of your skin tone. In my eyes, you can never have enough nude bras!

Black is Back. You also need at least two black bras for wearing under darker clothing, especially black. A nude bra, especially the edges of the cups, can show through black if the sweater or top is at all sheer. In cases like this, a plain black bra will work better!

BRA COLOR	TOP OR DRESS COLOR
Nude	Wear under any and every color, and the sheerest of fabrics!
White	Wear under colors only. Do not wear under white!
Black	Wear under black/navy.
Bright Colors	Wear under black/navy/other bright colors.
Patterned/Lace/ Multi-colored	Wear under black/navy/other bright colors. (*Caution*: If the color is dark but the fabric is thin or sheer, you may need a nude or less textured bra instead.)

A BRA FOR EVERY BODY TYPE

Your outfit shouldn't be the only thing flattering your figure. Your bra should be figure-flattering, too! The right bra can help create a more balanced silhouette under clothes. The first step, though, is knowing just what your "figure" is.

While there are many different theories for classifying female figures, for our purposes we'll use a common guideline that outlines four basic body types:

◀ Apple or upside-down triangle: Women with this body type tend to store fat around the midsection, making them rounder in the middle like an apple and creating a body shape that's broader on the top and narrower on the bottom like an upside-down triangle.

▶ Hourglass: Women with this body type look like hourglasses: evenly proportioned on top and bottom, with noticeable narrowing at the waist.

BRA FASHION FAST FACT

A 2005 study by researchers at North Carolina State University found that even though only about 8 percent of women are hourglass-shaped, clothing designers and manufacturers were still building clothes based on a slim version of that body type. Of the 6,000 women studied, nearly half were rectangles while just over 20 percent were pear-shaped. About 14 percent were apples or inverted triangles.

 Pear: Women with this body type are shaped just like the fruit, with a smaller curve on the top and a fuller curve on the bottom.

▶ Rectangle or banana: Women with this body type tend to be more muscular and athletic, and often do not have an especially defined waistline, creating a straighter silhouette.

Most women fall into one of these categories.

Certain bras enhance certain shapes better than others. The key is to choose a bra that evens out your proportions. For example, if you're larger on top, like an apple or upside-down triangle, you may want to look for a minimizing bra. If you're larger on the bottom, like a pear, you may want to look for a push-up bra with a little padding to balance out your wider hips.

In the chart on the next page, note your body type and what kind of bras you should be looking for.

BODY TYPE	WHAT TO LOOK FOR/ WHAT TO AVOID
Apple/ Inverted Triangle	Look For: minimizing bras (which will deemphasize your larger bust) Avoid: push-up and padded bras (which make you look even larger on top)
Hourglass	You can wear almost any bra; lucky you! But you might want to look for something that enhances your cleavage and further accentuates your hourglass shape.
Pear	Look For: push-up and padded bras (which will go a long way in balancing out your ample hips) Avoid: bralettes and minimizing bras (which compress and deemphasize your breasts)
Banana/Rectangle	Look For: cleavage-enhancing bra with wide-set straps, like balconettes (which will narrow your shoulders and feminize your figure) Avoid: minimizing bras or compression type sports bras (which will make your shoulders and chest appear broader)

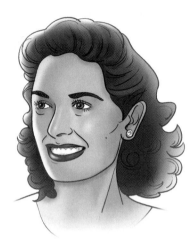

BRA FASHION
FAST FACT
Need a little extra oomph in
a strapless gown? Insert gel
pads, also known as cutlets,
into your bra for an added,
natural-looking boost.

"Forty pictures I was in and all
I remember is 'What kind of
bra will you be wearing today,
honey?' That was always the
area of big decision—from
the neck to the navel."
—Donna Reed

To sum up what we've learned in this chapter: Make note of your body type, stock up on black and nude bras, opt for versatile styles that will take you from a day at the office to your best friend's wedding with just a switch of the straps, and while comfort is key, don't forget to snag a few sexy styles, too. You'll be sure to have the right bra for every occasion—and every outfit!

five

Your Bra

and

Your Body

REMEMBER THE FAMOUS BROOKE SHIELDS COMMERCIAL WHERE SHE proclaimed, "Nothing gets between me and my Calvin's?" Forget jeans. Nothing gets between you and your bra, literally. It's the closest thing to your body at all times . . . and the article of clothing that's perhaps *most* affected by changes to your body.

Our bodies don't look the same at ten as they do at forty, so why would our breasts? According to a study of 500 women conducted by www.myintimacy.com, the average woman's breasts will "change shape, size, and distribution at least six times during the course of her life." Our breasts are constantly changing. Though the most dramatic changes tend to occur at puberty, we experience a bevy of body changes throughout our lifetimes that can affect what we need from our bras. That's why it's important to understand what these changes are, and how our breasts can support us through them, both physically and emotionally.

In this chapter, we'll look at seven common changes our breasts go through:

▶ Puberty

▶ Pregnancy and breastfeeding

▶ Weight loss or gain

▶ Mastectomy

▶ Breast augmentation and other surgery to the breasts

▶ Menstrual cycle, menopause, and other hormonal fluctuations

▶ Aging

PUBERTY

At the onset of puberty—generally between the ages of nine and sixteen—a girl typically gets her period, starts to grow body hair, and begins to develop breasts. She'll often also start wearing a bra during this time, even if she doesn't yet have a whole lot to put in it.

Whether because it's more socially acceptable (all her friends are wearing one) or her breasts have actually begun to develop, you'll want to get her what's typically known as a "training bra." Training bras come in sizes that are smaller than an A-cup (such as AAA and AA), and are generally wireless and made of comfortable, stretchy fabrics such as cotton blends. For young girls who

are blossoming a bit larger right off the bat, you may want to skip directly to a soft-cup bra such as the CC Girl Seamless Pull-Over Day Bra, which is made specifically for girls who are going through puberty (you can find it at www.dotgirlproducts.com, a site that caters to and educates about a girl's firsts: first periods, first bras, and more!). A compression-style sports bra, which comes in sizes small, medium, and large, is also a suitable alternative to a training bra. You can use your child's clothing sizes as a guideline.

If you have a pre-teen or teen who is about to go through puberty or who is currently in the middle of it, be sure to help

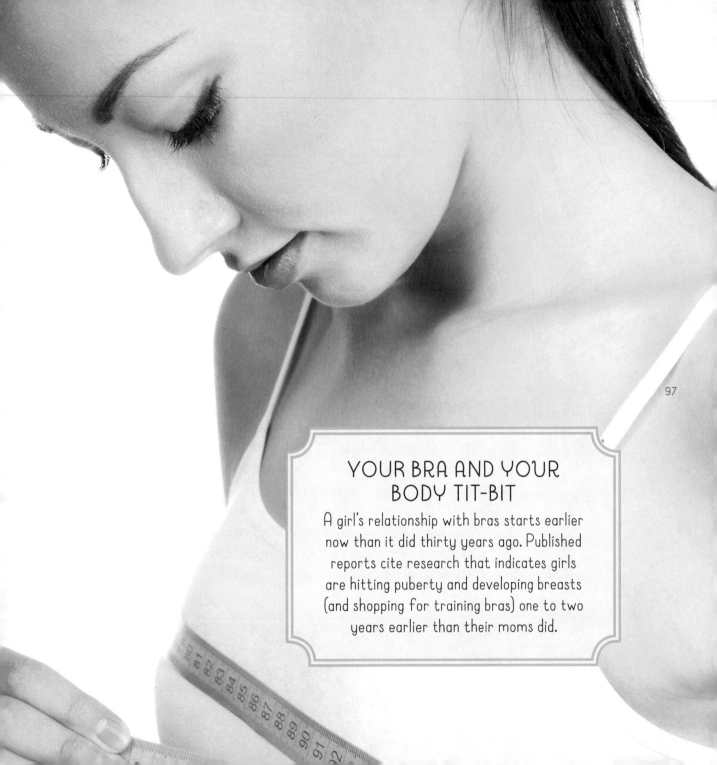

YOUR BRA AND YOUR BODY TIT-BIT

A girl's relationship with bras starts earlier now than it did thirty years ago. Published reports cite research that indicates girls are hitting puberty and developing breasts (and shopping for training bras) one to two years earlier than their moms did.

IT'S NOT JUST ABOUT THE JOCK STRAP

A 2016 study in the *Journal of Adolescent Health* found that girls are dropping out of sports and skipping gym class around the time they hit puberty. Why do researchers believe this is happening? In a study of 2,089 girls aged eleven to eighteen, nearly three-quarters of them had at least one breast-related complaint when it came to exercising. 90 percent of girls studied said they wanted to know more about breasts in general, and nearly half wanted to know more about bras for proper "sports support." This means that pediatricians, parents, coaches, and health educators can do a better job of talking to young girls about the changes to their body and how it can affect physical activity.

her through this process by educating her and supporting her as much as she needs. Mistakes in a girl's early bra-wearing days can be very damaging to her emotional health. As a teenager, I was mocked in school for not wearing a bra when everyone else had already begun wearing one (I didn't need one yet!), and it's something I still remember as an adult! Some parents believe there's a certain age a girl should start wearing one, while others hit the stores as early as the first appearance of breast buds.

The best way to help her through this important milestone is to take her to a department store or lingerie store for an expert bra fitting (and while you're at it, get one for yourself, too!). She will have to do this many more times in her life, so this will help her become comfortable with it early on and alleviate the embarrassment factor as she grows and matures.

One thing I hear from moms of tweens and teens all the time is that their girls are developed to double-Ds and the only bras (and swimsuits) on the market that fit them are overtly sexy because they're marketed to more mature women! My advice is to take your teen to a department store with lots of options, and opt for a basic molded cup t-shirt bra with full coverage cups. Skip anything with padding, push-up, sexy print, or lace detailing. Even if they develop early, we want our kids to stay kids, right?

PREGNANCY AND BREASTFEEDING

Pregnancy, quite possibly the biggest milestone in a woman's life, also takes the biggest toll on her body—including her breasts. The rapid weight gain and loss and the breastfeeding that often follows can cause everything from sagging to volume loss. "Predicting how a woman's breasts will change with pregnancy is a task for a genie with a crystal ball," says Dr. Garth Fisher, renowned Beverly Hills plastic surgeon, *Extreme Makeover* star, and author of the DVD series *The Naked Truth about Plastic Surgery.* "In general, pregnancy and nursing will cause the breast to engorge, stretch, and [then] droop or deflate."

The breasts are often the first part of the body to be affected by pregnancy, and your bra size—and type of bra you need—will inevitably change, both during and after pregnancy. According to "The New Moms' Nursing Bra Guide," an article on www.ezinearticles.com, during pregnancy and breastfeeding, women generally go up at least one band size *and* one cup size, thanks to swollen breasts and a ribcage that's growing to accommodate your growing baby. Some women have reported going through dozens of bras in those nine months alone. During my first pregnancy, which occurred while I was writing this book, I went up two full cup sizes in the first trimester!

Your maternity bra needs will be dependent on how much (and how often) your body changes during pregnancy. And it's more important than ever to wear the right size when pregnant, because an incorrect fit can put pressure on your sensitive breasts, causing mastitis (an inflammation of the mammary glands) and plugged milk ducts. Plus, breasts are often very tender and sore during and after pregnancy, and a supportive bra will limit potentially painful movement. Providing proper support will also prevent unnecessary strain on your neck and shoulders from heavier, swollen breasts. So while you're shopping for maternity clothes, you'll also want to invest in a good "maternity" bra. These are generally soft-cup bras in a comfy fabric like cotton, often with light padding for sore, tender nipples and wider straps for added support.

At the end of your pregnancy, if you plan to nurse you will want to switch to a nursing bra, which has cups that open from the front to allow easy access for breastfeeding. There are four different

YOUR BRA AND YOUR BODY TIT-BIT

If during pregnancy your band is getting too tight but the cups are still fitting well, you can try bra extenders. They hook on to the back of your current bras to add inches of comfort (especially useful when you get to the point where your bra band is resting on the top of your belly!).

types of nursing bras, each one providing a different method for allowing the baby access to your breast. The first fastens between the cups in the front. The second has zippers that sit under each cup. The third fastens at the straps, allowing you to pull the cups down. The last has a crossover design in the front that allows you to just slip your breast out. Just choose the design that you will be most comfortable with!

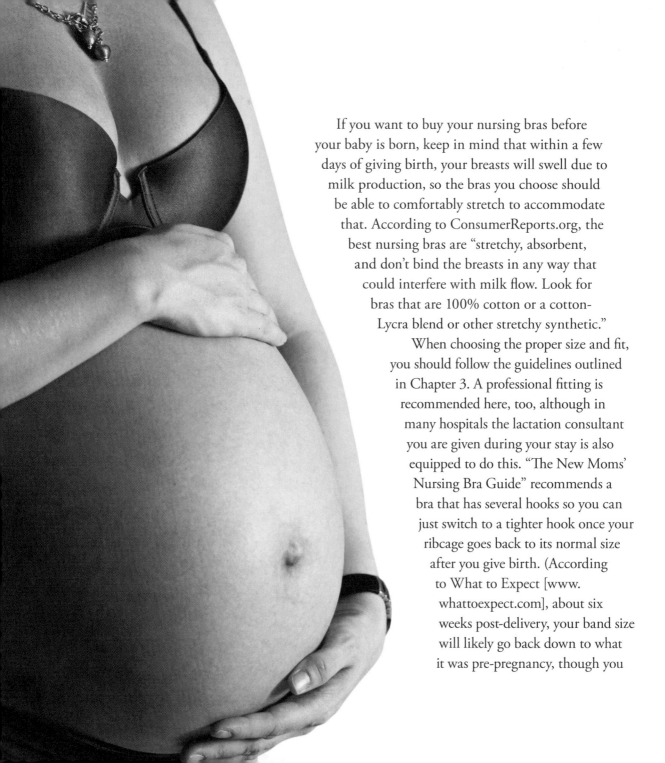

If you want to buy your nursing bras before your baby is born, keep in mind that within a few days of giving birth, your breasts will swell due to milk production, so the bras you choose should be able to comfortably stretch to accommodate that. According to ConsumerReports.org, the best nursing bras are "stretchy, absorbent, and don't bind the breasts in any way that could interfere with milk flow. Look for bras that are 100% cotton or a cotton-Lycra blend or other stretchy synthetic."

When choosing the proper size and fit, you should follow the guidelines outlined in Chapter 3. A professional fitting is recommended here, too, although in many hospitals the lactation consultant you are given during your stay is also equipped to do this. "The New Moms' Nursing Bra Guide" recommends a bra that has several hooks so you can just switch to a tighter hook once your ribcage goes back to its normal size after you give birth. (According to What to Expect [www. whattoexpect.com], about six weeks post-delivery, your band size will likely go back down to what it was pre-pregnancy, though you may remain about a cup size larger. Everyone is different!) The Body Silk Seamless Nursing Bra by Bravado! Designs is actually designed to fit several band and cup sizes to allow for your body's fluctuations during this time.

During breastfeeding, you may want to avoid bras that have an underwire, as one that is too tight can restrict the milk ducts and cause serious complications. In the absence of an underwire, however, the straps and cups will end up taking on more of the support responsibilities, so look for a bra with wider straps and consider investing in attachable shoulder strap pads to alleviate any digging in. You may also want to opt for a nursing bra with some slight padding. I have friends who have learned the hard way that,

otherwise, milk can leak from your breasts and cause some embarrassment when you're wearing a thin top.

When trying on a nursing bra, you'll want to not only check for comfort and fit but also whether the cups are easy to open when you have your hungry newborn in your arms. You'll have plenty of options to choose from (ConsumerReports.org did a review of several of them), including athletic styles that are extra supportive, styles for sleeping in, and even some built into tank tops. For the best selection of maternity and nursing bras, visit stores with inventory especially for expectant moms, like the national chain Destination Maternity (their staff is also trained in fitting).

WEIGHT GAIN OR LOSS

· ·

When you gain weight, your breasts can stretch and grow along with the rest of your body. When you lose weight, your breasts may lose volume, too. Every woman's body is different: Some women don't lose any weight at all in their breasts when they drop pounds, making their breasts seem proportionately larger, and others lose weight in their breasts first. The best thing to do after any shift in weight is get re-fitted; even if the volume of your breasts hasn't changed, your band size may have!

Changes in weight can cause more than just changes in breast size. When you gain and then lose weight, your skin—which has

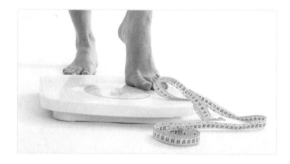

stretched to accommodate the additional weight—may still be stretched out. In the breasts, this can result in a decrease in fullness and firmness. A push-up or padded bra, or the use of cutlets, can aid in giving the appearance of volume and firmness back to your breasts.

POST-MASTECTOMY

Unfortunately, most of us know someone who has had to undergo a breast removal procedure, or mastectomy. This is usually done as a treatment for (or in some cases for the prevention of) breast cancer, which 1 in 8 women will get in her lifetime, according to American Cancer Society statistics.

If you have to undergo a mastectomy, whether or not the procedure involves an immediate reconstruction, you will generally want to purchase a special post-mastectomy bra (though women should wear post-surgical garments for six to eight weeks after surgery before switching to even a post-mastectomy bra). Post-mastectomy bras are usually made of soft, breathable cotton, have specially designed straps to prevent "cup bounce," and are adjustable for ease of movement and to keep from irritating the surgery site. While these bras are often designed with pockets to hold breast forms, or prostheses, in place, a pocketed bra is not absolutely necessary. The benefit of a pocketed bra is that it helps absorb moisture between the chest and breast form and also keeps the prosthesis from slipping out of place.

Some companies are going an extra step to make post-surgical bras more comfortable for women. Amoena's Hanna Collection is

106

YOUR BRA AND YOUR BODY TIT-BIT

Early detection of breast cancer can not only prevent you from having to undergo a mastectomy, it can also save your life. The American Cancer Society says women over forty should have a mammogram—an X-ray of the breast—every year. Women at high risk (those with a family history or who have been diagnosed with the so-called "breast cancer gene") should start screening as early as age thirty. It's also important to do monthly self-exams at home so if you feel any unusual lumps you can bring them to the attention of your doctor.

one of the industry's first to offer camisoles and bras infused with vitamin E and aloe to ease discomfort and promote healing after breast surgery. The company also has specially trained fit specialists on hand to help breast cancer patients find the best bra to meet their needs at www.amoena.com.

Some women undergo post-mastectomy breast reconstruction through the use of "tissue expanders," which are temporary saline implants placed at the site or sites where breast tissue is removed. Through a series of doctor's visits over several months, saline is pumped into the implant, gradually stretching the skin. In this case, you might wear a different bra size through every stage of the expansion, so be prepared to get re-fitted every time.

Vera Garofalo, post-mastectomy expert and program manager of Hope's Boutique at the James Cancer Hospital and Solove Research Institute in Dublin, Ohio, strongly recommends visiting a mastectomy fitter who has been certified by the American Board for Certification in Orthotics, Prosthetics, and Pedorthics. You can find one near you by visiting their website at www.abcop.org/Mastectomy_Fitter.asp.

Meanwhile, here are Vera's tips for shopping for post-mastectomy bras:

▶ The band of the bra should hook so it fits comfortably snug just like with a regular bra. Having the correct band size is especially important to prevent the bra from shifting or riding up, since this can dislodge or displace the prosthesis. You are trying to simulate the natural breast, which, unlike the prosthesis, is attached to your body and cannot move. Also, when the prosthesis does not stay secure, it can cause rubbing at the surgery site, causing extra sensitivity, and continually pulling at your bra if it is shifting or riding up will only increase that discomfort.

▶ The straps should be adjusted so that each breast and/or prosthesis is held securely and at a comfortable level. Straps should fit snugly without cutting into the shoulders; you should be able to get one finger under the strap. You may want to look for padded straps for added comfort or opt for separate, attachable strap pads. The prosthesis will inevitably differ in weight from the natural breast,

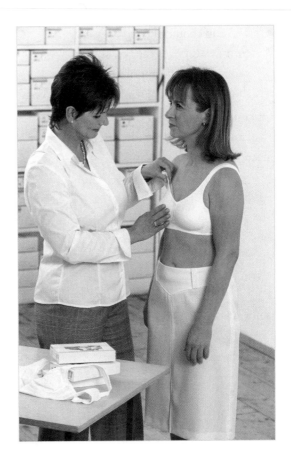

Woman getting fitted for a post-mastectomy bra.

107

and adjusting the straps is crucial for achieving symmetry and keeping the prosthesis secure.

> ▶ The cup should fit smoothly and completely cover the breast tissue *and* surgical area. For optimum comfort, it should hug the chest without any gaping.

Of course, any and all options and care for post surgery should be discussed with and monitored by your doctor.

BREAST AUGMENTATION AND OTHER SURGERY TO THE BREASTS

Millions of women are opting to go under the knife for bigger—or smaller—boobs. In fact, for the first time since the American Society of Plastic Surgeons began compiling statistics, breast augmentation was found to be the most popular cosmetic surgical procedure, with hundreds of thousands of women undergoing the procedure each and every year. There are also many women who opt to undergo breast reduction surgery, often because their breasts are so large or heavy that it causes them physical pain. In each case, finding the right bra afterward can involve special challenges.

If you undergo breast augmentation surgery, or an enlargement of the breasts through the use of implants, you can expect to wear a post-surgical bra for four to six weeks after surgery. In some cases, this is a compression-style bra with a strap on top that is used to push the implants downward and keep them in place. In others, you may be given a soft bra that resembles a sports bra (or an actual sports bra!) instead. Which bra you receive depends on the surgeon, the incisions, and the extent of the enlargement. Most doctors determine the best post-operative bra on a case-by-case basis. After

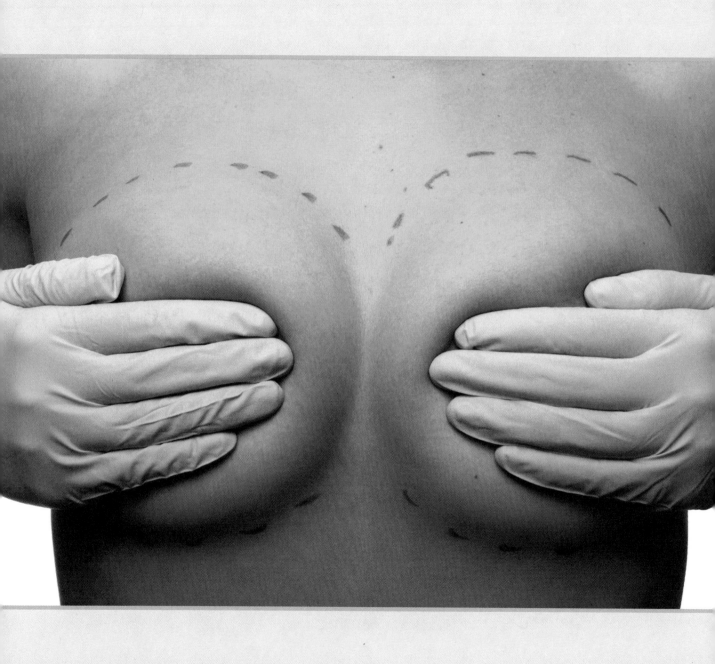

this four- to six-week period, usually the first thing you'll want to do is dash out to the lingerie store to shop for your new, improved size. But figuring out bra size isn't any easier for breast augmentation patients than it is for anyone else.

It's a misconception that your doctor can tell you your new bra size based on the size of the implants inserted. We've all heard the women on makeover shows say, "Make me a C cup," or "I want to be a D," but every doctor I've spoken to tells me this is unrealistic. Implants come in many sizes, and none of them correspond to cup size. Implant sizes are named by the volume of solution (either saline or silicone) that the implant holds, often measured in CCs, or cubic centimeters. And as we already know, cup sizes are determined in proportion to band sizes. So a doctor certainly can't tell you for sure that your new size will be a C-cup.

As always, your first step should be to get a professional fitting to determine your new size. But it's best to wait until the swelling has gone down (unless you plan on buying new bras—*again*—once it does). When this happens all depends on your

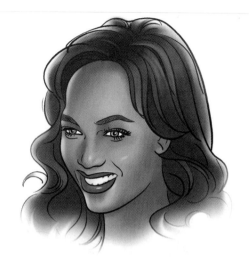

111

"I am totally against plastic surgery. A lot of people think I have breast implants because I have the biggest boobs in the business. But I was a 34C when I was seventeen . . . They stay up when I wear a push-up bra. But if people could see me when I come home and take off my bra, how could they think these are fake?"
—Tyra Banks

body. While doctors say swelling can start to subside in as little as two weeks, you won't be at your new true size and shape until at least six to eight weeks. For some women, it can take up to three months.

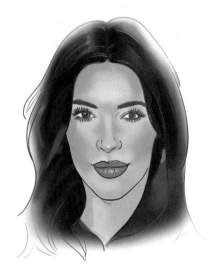

"I have had a size C since I was eleven years old! One day I will definitely get a lift, but I am waiting until after I have kids. Until then, I rely on a great supportive bra!"
—Kim Kardashian (2008)

Once you have been fitted and purchased new bras, it's a good idea to take them to your doctor to make sure they won't interfere with the healing process in any way. Even after the swelling subsides, your breasts are still healing and can continue to do so for months.

Speaking of healing, if your surgery involved incisions around the nipple or an added procedure such as a breast lift that involves multiple incisions, you'll want to look for a bra in a soft, "non-scratchy" fabric like cotton so you won't risk irritating them. If your incisions are in the breast fold, as they are in many augmentations, underwire could irritate them, so you may want to stick to a bra without underwire until the incisions are completely healed.

There is a common myth that wearing a push-up or underwire bra can harm augmented breasts or cause your implants to shift. Some doctors will even argue the same. But I consulted with New York–based plastic surgeon Dr. C. Andrew Salzberg, the self-proclaimed pioneer of the One-Stage Breast Reconstruction procedure (in which women who undergo a mastectomy receive a reconstruction in

HOLLYWOOD BREASTS

Breasts come in all shapes and sizes, yet plastic surgeons say more and more women are asking for round, unnaturally shaped breasts. Is Hollywood to blame? "I believe the craze for 'round Hollywood breasts' started with Pamela Anderson and the *Baywatch* days," says plastic surgeon Dr. Garth Fisher. "Some of the most visualized breasts on television were round and oversized and many of the first implants were made in that shape." According to most doctors, natural breasts tend to be shaped more like a teardrop.

Today implants are being made in all shapes and sizes so a woman can have whatever she desires. Silicone gel implants are a popular choice and can help give breasts a more natural look and feel compared to the saline variety. There are also bras that create the much-sought "round" implant look. Through strategically placed pads in the lower part of the cup, this bra helps push together and round out the breasts, creating a very spherical appearance and covetable cleavage.

the same operation), and he disputes this. "There is no reason you can't wear any bra you want and no medical proof to support claims that underwire will harm the implant," says Salzberg. "The only thing that can cause the implant to move is if the internal 'pocket' that holds the breast implant is too big or, over time, the muscle comes up, causing the implant to slide down—not a bra." Ill-fitting underwire that is not positioned properly in your breast fold and is digging into your breast tissue, however, can certainly cause pain and discomfort. Many doctors do advise avoiding underwire altogether for at least the first month or two if your surgery involved incisions in the folds of the breasts. You want to avoid anything that might rub against the incision site, because it can cause irritation and possibly make the scars worse.

One other thing to keep in mind when buying post-augmentation bras: Implants are often also wider than natural breasts, so you may need to look for a fuller-coverage cup than you're used to.

What if your surgery involved a reduction in breast size? According to Dr.

Andrew Kleinman, a plastic surgeon in Rye Brook, New York, post-surgical bras for breast reduction patients don't differ that much from augmentation patients'. However, the breast reduction patient usually "will wear this bra for a week or two and then is usually able to switch to any bra that is comfortable and doesn't irritate any incision sites."

Because every reduction patient is different—every patient has a different amount of breast tissue removed, plus age, skin texture, and whether or not the patient has had children can all be factors—the number of bras you can expect to go through post-surgery is hard to predict, too. "Swelling does change over the course of a few months and the new shape of the breasts has to settle over the course of a few months, too," says Dr. Kleinman. "How long this process takes is very dependent on the surgical technique used and the patient. It is not uncommon after a substantial reduction for the size and shape to change for up to a year." That means lots of bra fittings—and lots of bras. But, Dr. Kleinman adds, most patients will be fit into a bra that will be "fairly appropriate for the long-term" after about three months.

Perhaps the hardest thing for reduction patients to grasp is that the size of their breasts is not the only thing that will change after surgery—the shape will, too. "With a reduction, you are not just changing the size of the breasts to make them smaller; you're also restoring the position of the breast to a more normal position since women with very large breasts tend to experience a lot of sagging," Dr. Kleinman notes. So you're looking at not just size, but position and shape changes, too.

Reduction patients also have much different scarring patterns than augmentation patients. Scars can range from a small line around the areola, to a "lollipop" shape on the breast, to an "anchor" shape—which can make it more difficult to find a bra that won't irritate your incision site. "It's important to find a bra that's comfortable and doesn't irritate any of the incisions while they are healing. A bra that rubs against the incision sites can cause skin sores, so you want to avoid that at all costs. That is even more important than finding the proper fit after surgery. If you can find a fit that's close enough, and it feels comfortable, then you are in the right bra."

Whether you're having a breast enlargement or a reduction, Dr. Kleinman says, you'll want to keep in mind that the shape of your breasts will change over the years in slightly different ways than natural breasts would. "Just like a woman who has larger breasts will sag faster than a woman with smaller breasts, women with breasts that have been operated on will notice different changes than those who have un-augmented breasts. Healing is not a static thing with these procedures; it's dynamic. So you'll notice that you'll be changing the style of bra you like and wear every couple of years."

MENSTRUAL CYCLE, MENOPAUSE, AND OTHER HORMONAL FLUCTUATIONS

••

Ah, hormones. They are always messing everything up for us gals, right? And we have to deal with them not just during puberty, pregnancy, and menopause, but each and every month!

There are plenty of reasons your hormones can fluctuate (two of which—puberty and pregnancy—we've talked about already), but let's start with the most frequent: your period. During your period, swelling breasts can cause your bra size to increase up to one full cup size! Accordingly, it's good to keep at least one bra on hand that's a bit more "full coverage" to accommodate this change. You may even

want to purchase a bra or two specifically for that one week out of the month. Many women I know also switch to a bra with softer cups during this time to avoid irritating sensitive nipples.

Perhaps the biggest hormonal changes happen during menopause. Between hot flashes, decreased sex drive, and other menopausal symptoms, you also have to deal with changing breasts. According to the National Cancer Institute, "when you stop having periods at the onset of menopause, your hormone levels drop, and your breast tissue becomes less dense and more fatty." This can lead to increased sagging and the need for a bra that provides a little more lift, such as a push-up bra. However, there is no research to support the idea that you need any kind of "special" bra during this time—though because of hot flashes and sweating, you may want to choose bras in light, breathable fabrics.

There are other things besides our period and menopause that can cause water retention and affect hormone levels in a woman's body, like birth control, hormone replacement therapy, and other medications, and that can lead an increase in breast size

of up to one cup. Being on the pill alone can send your hormones into overdrive— the pill mimics the hormonal changes that occur during pregnancy and can cause your breasts to expand. In fact, the increase in average breast size over the past two decades has been attributed at least in part to the estrogen in birth controls pills (along with poor eating habits and increased obesity, and of course the popularity of implants). It's important that if you notice any change, you get re-fitted to ensure you are still wearing the proper size.

AGING

Just like our faces, our breasts can show our age. It's safe to assume that all women know aging has adverse effects on their breasts. Gravity is perhaps the worst culprit. Paired with the loss of skin elasticity that comes with age, gravity makes sagging over time inevitable. Add to that the body changes most women experience during their lives— pregnancy, weight loss and gain, etc.—and it's clear that the breasts take quite a beating! As a result, they can end up not just sitting lower, but actually changing shape and size entirely.

Unfortunately, there has been no solid evidence that suggests you can do anything

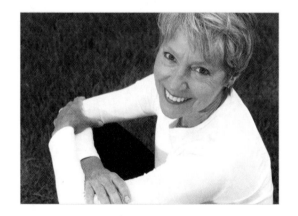

to prevent sagging. Some people say sleeping in your bra or constantly wearing an underwire will help, but others argue that wearing a bra *causes* sagging, because

YOUR BRA AND YOUR BODY TIT-BIT

There are some handy dandy gadgets on the market that can help combat the effects of aging. Try Bralief or Strap-Mate, both of which help boost the lift your bra provides by pulling the straps together in the back. Not only will this make your breasts appear younger and perkier, it will also keep pesky straps from falling down.

our breasts are made up of ligaments and those ligaments aren't able to retain their strength when a bra is doing their job for them. (We'll be exploring these ideas more in-depth in Chapter 6.)

But once your girls begin to head south, you don't have to go under the knife—the right bra can turn back the hands of time. Simply finding a bra that fits correctly can take years and pounds off of your appearance by boosting your breasts back up to their proper position. If you'd like some added oomph, you can always opt for a push-up bra or a bra with some padding. Many women think they are "too old" for a push-up bra, but this is not the case! The only number you should pay attention to when it comes to your bra choice is your band size. You have a right to perkier breasts at any age!

It's time to separate the myths from the facts! Is your bra bad for your health? Can it *cause* cancer, as some believe? Continue on to Chapter 6 to find out more.

six

Breast Rx

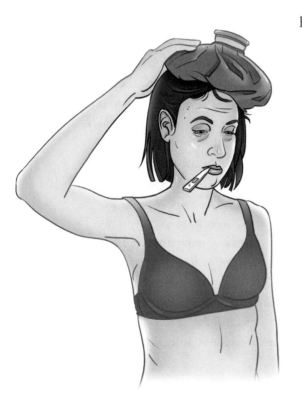

CAN YOUR BRA BE BAD FOR YOUR HEALTH? ALL YOU HAVE TO DO IS GOOGLE the words "bra" and "cancer" and thousands of posts will pop up. Believe it or not, there is a debate about whether your bra can *cause* cancer. The subject has even been studied and researched.

As you'll learn in this chapter, that's not the only health concern surrounding bras. The wrong bra can cause problems both inside and out—everything from bad posture and skin irritations to muscle strain, migraines, and even indigestion! Your bra can even negatively affect your ability to *breathe* properly. And besides affecting how we *feel*, the wrong bra can also affect how we *look*—not just temporarily but, some say, permanently.

There's a lot of disagreement out there about bras' impact on our health. There are people who believe underwire harms ultra-sensitive breast tissue; others think it's necessary for proper support. There are some who say wearing a bra contributes to sagging breasts, and others who believe a bra helps *prevent* sagging. As you continue reading this chapter, you'll learn what's true and what's not, and how to separate bra myths from the bra facts.

STRAIN

As if stress and everyday life don't put enough strain on our bodies, we have to worry about our bras doing it, too! The one thing that everyone seems to agree on is that an improperly fitted bra can cause muscle strain. If you're feeling tension in your shoulders, upper back, neck, and head, your bra could be to blame—it may not be giving you the support you need. And when you experience upper body strain, it affects your ability to stand up straight, causing poor posture. Fuller-breasted women carry even more weight on their shoulders (literally), so getting a fit that prevents strain is that much more important.

Too-tight straps and back bands can also cause another problem: headaches. "If [your bra] is too tight around the back, it can compress the muscles of the upper back, which will then compress a nerve going up toward the scalp, triggering tension and headaches," says Dr. Dave E. David, a Massachusetts-based OB/GYN.

These problems can be seen as well as felt. If your bra is leaving any kind of marks, either around your ribcage or on your shoulders, it's putting a strain on your body (not to mention irritating your skin). As we mentioned in Chapter 3, you'll want to make sure you can fit at least one to two fingers underneath your band at all times. And to reduce pressure on your shoulders and the potential for strain, you can opt for wider straps (at least a half-inch or more in width) and bras with underwire that offer more support in the cups.

Bras can also put strain on your lungs. Believe it or not, a bra that's too tight can affect your ability to *breathe*! Patricia Bowden-Luccardi is a breathing therapist and educator for the Radiance Wellness Center in Hudson, New York, and lecturer on "The Power of Breath" at Massachusetts' Canyon Ranch Resort and Spa. "When your bra is too tight, it inhibits proper breathing," says Luccardi. "And when your breathing is constricted, scientific evidence links that to cardiovascular disease, high blood pressure, and other symptoms like gas, bloating, and acid reflux." The website Optimal Breathing (www.breathing.com) makes the analogy that trying to breathe deeply when your chest and back muscles are restricted by tight-fitting clothing (like a too-tight bra) is like "trying to blow up a 5-quart balloon inside a 3- to 4-quart bottle." A better-fitting bra will not just make you look and feel better, it will help you breathe a little easier, too.

ARE THERE WAYS TO INCREASE BREAST SIZE "NATURALLY"?

· ·

We've all seen the infomercials about exercise, massage, creams, and "herbal supplements," and heard the middle-school exercise myths ("we must, we must, we must increase our busts!"). But short of hormones or gaining weight, can we really increase the size of our breasts? In short, no. Weight training can strengthen the underlying chest muscles, but that won't necessarily make breasts themselves larger. As for herbal supplements, there is no medical evidence to support the claims that these really work.

An external "tissue expander" system known as Brava (www.mybrava. com) has shown promising results in some women. The company claims women who follow the regimen can boost their breasts by as much of a full cup size. The regimen? Wearing a battery-powered, vacuum-like bra device (torture device?) eleven hours a day for at least ten consecutive weeks. Ouch!

SICKNESS

It's scary to think that a bra could actually make us *sick*. But some researchers believe it has the potential to do just that. The controversial 1996 book *Dressed to Kill: The Link Between Breast Cancer and Bras*, by Sydney Ross Singer and Soma Grismaijer, outlined the findings of a study they conducted of nearly 5,000 women in which they claim to have found a link between bras and breast cancer (although it's important to note that no other studies have duplicated the book's findings, so the information in it should be taken with a grain of salt). The authors say they discovered that women who wear tight-fitting bras (bras that are tight enough to put pressure on the lymphatic system, an internal network of vessels and nodes that flush waste from the body) twenty-four hours a day are 125 times more likely to get breast cancer than women who do not wear bras at all, and women who wear bras more than twelve hours a day increase their chances of getting breast cancer dramatically.

Much like tight bras can press against our upper body and restrict our breathing, Singer and Grismaijer say, bras (specifically those with underwire) press against our breast tissue, restricting circulation and blood flow to the breasts and causing a

> ## BREAST RX MYTH DEBUNKED
> Breast cancer is said to be more common in Western cultures where women have been wearing bras for more than a century. This has added fuel to the fiery debate that bras contribute to causing breast cancer. However, the National Research Center for Women and Families says that there are more plausible explanations for this, such as the fact that in less-developed countries, people have less access to medical care and therefore cases of breast cancer often go undiagnosed. Other researchers suggest that a difference in nutrition—like the higher saturated fat content in the Western diet—may better explain the difference. People also tend to not live as long in these areas, and since breast cancer strikes more frequently in older women, these countries' rates would be lower regardless of whether their inhabitants wore bras.

malfunction of the lymphatic system. When the lymphatic system isn't functioning properly, it cannot drain waste, trapping toxins in our breasts. This causes the toxins to settle in breast tissue and become reabsorbed, causing cancer.

Critics of this book dispute the way the "study" was conducted, stating that (among other issues) additional variables weren't taken into consideration, such as other known risk factors for breast cancer. Debate continues to rage on.

Before you toss your bra, think about this: While almost all American women wear bras, according to the American Cancer Society just one out of every eight of us will be diagnosed with breast cancer at some point in her lifetime. But if you're concerned, you can simply opt to not wear a bra for part of the day (most likely while you're lounging around at home) or switch to a more comfortable, non-binding one altogether, such as a simple cotton bra without an underwire. For most women, the benefits of wearing a bra far outweigh the potential "risks" described in these claims—which is probably why the bra business is still booming, despite the release of Singer and Grismaijer's book more than a decade ago.

Another controversial claim against bras is that those allegedly contaminated with the chemical formaldehyde are giving some women persistent skin rashes and severe discomfort. Formaldehyde is found in many everyday products as a preservative but has been tagged a "probable carcinogen" or cancer-causing agent by the Environmental Protection Agency and is a known allergen. It's also illegal for use in textiles in this country. There have been no definitive answers on whether the bras in question were actually contaminated with formaldehyde or whether formaldehyde was the culprit in the women's illness.

One sickness that *has* been proven to come in part from your bra is mastitis, the inflammation of breast tissues due to obstruction and infection of the milk ducts. Mastitis can occur in breastfeeding women who wear a nursing bra that is too tight and puts pressure on the milk ducts (though mastitis can be caused by other factors as well, such as irregular breastfeeding or sleeping on your tummy for long periods of time). A looser, more comfortable bra with flaps that doesn't press against the area around your nipple is a good option to help prevent bra-induced mastitis. You can also talk to a lactation consultant if you're concerned. And of course, any and all infections should be treated by your doctor.

Your bra can also make your skin sick. A combination of sweat and your bra's fabric rubbing against the breast (especially if the bra doesn't fit right) can cause a mild, itchy fungal infection. According to Manhattan plastic surgeon Dr. Matthew Schulman, "rashes and fungal infections can develop on the skin on and around a woman's breasts if she's not wearing a material that breathes." This is particularly important for larger-breasted women or women who work out (and sweat) in their bras, and hot and humid conditions can make infection more likely,

129

but this kind of skin irritation can happen to anyone. Switching to a natural fiber bra (such as cotton) can help you avoid infection—the fabric will breathe better and so be less likely to cause conditions in which fungus can grow. A hydrocortisone or antifungal cream applied to the skin on and under the breast can help treat a rash if one has already developed, but be sure to also wash your bras in hot water to prevent re-infection.

SAGGING

Gravity: What was considered a scientific breakthrough when Sir Isaac Newton first discovered it has, three centuries later, become the enemy of women everywhere. Bras are designed to oppose it, by holding our breasts up as the forces of gravity pull them down. But even the best of push-up bras can't stop our gals from sagging over time. So what really causes sagging? And why does it happen to some women earlier than others? Can it be made worse by breastfeeding? By not wearing a bra? By *wearing* a bra?

Some researchers say that wearing a bra can prevent breasts from developing (or strengthening) their own internal support structure, which contributes to sagging. But many doctors disagree. "Overall, gravity plays the biggest role in breast sagging," says Las Vegas plastic surgeon Dr. Samir Pancholi. "We've all heard about the ninety-year-old woman who had small, perky breasts when she was younger and now that gravity has gotten a hold of them, they aren't perky anymore."

According to Dr. Matthew Schulman, sagging mainly results from three things: "Loss of skin support or elastin; loss of the internal supporting structure of the breast—known as Cooper's Ligaments—

which serve as an 'internal bra'; and involution or loss of breast tissue with age, weight changes, and pregnancy."

Pancholi elaborates on the factors that contribute to sagging:

Pregnancy: "As the breasts increase in size, the skin stretches. Many times, the skin will stretch farther than its elastic fibers can handle. When this happens, it's like a rubber band that has been stretched out for too long—it simply won't spring back."

Aging: "As women age, the different elements of the environment [affect] the integrity of the skin. This causes the skin's structural components

to break down and allows it to stretch, causing sagging."

Augmentation: "When women come in for surgery to enlarge their breasts, the bigger the implant, the more the skin gets stretched out, and it's like the rubber band effect all over again. These elastic fibers can only hang on for so long before they allow the breasts to start sagging. This is compounded by implants that are placed above the muscle as opposed to underneath it. [An implant placed above the muscle] only has the skin and breast tissue to keep it in place— pretty stretchy tissue and not the strongest elements of the body."

132

BREAST RX MYTH DEBUNKED

Does sleeping in a bra help prevent sagging? Doctors say there is no evidence to support such claims. Just sleep in whatever makes you feel most comfortable!

DOES BREASTFEEDING CAUSE SAGGING?

· ·

While pregnancy surely contributes to breast sagging, a 2007 study dispels the myth that *breastfeeding* alone does. The American Academy of Plastic Surgeons found that while 55 percent of women studied noticed an adverse change in the shape of their breasts following pregnancy, none reported any changes after breastfeeding for a duration of two to twenty-five months. The same study also found that it wasn't the swift weight gain and loss associated with pregnancy that determined whether a woman's breasts sagged. Instead, it was factors like the woman's pre-pregnancy BMI or body mass index, the number of pregnancies she'd had, whether or not she had large breasts before pregnancy, her age, and whether or not she was a smoker.

CAN EXERCISING YOUR CHEST MUSCLES HELP PREVENT SAGGING?

Yes and no. Since our breasts are made up of tissue and ligaments (not muscle), there is really no way bench pressing will help keep breasts themselves firm. However, for some women, beefing up the pec muscles *beneath* the breasts can help create the appearance of perkier breasts!

Here are three potentially boob-boosting exercises you can add to your gym routine:

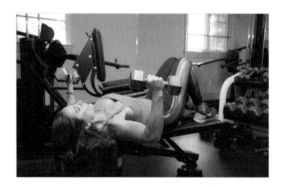 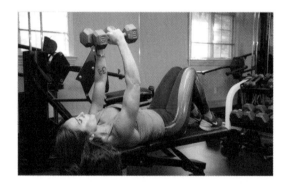

Pectoral Flies: Lie on your back on a flat bench and, holding dumbbells, extend your arms into the air with palms facing in. Keeping elbows slightly bent, lower weights to slightly higher than the shoulder line. Squeezing the chest, bring weights back up to starting position. Aim to do 3 sets of 12–15 reps.

Here's an extra tit-bit: Doing this exercise on an incline bench, as opposed to a flat bench, can potentially fight that pesky overhang around the armpits known as bra bulge!

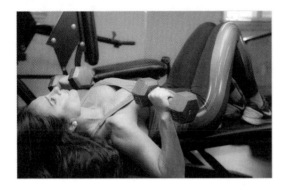
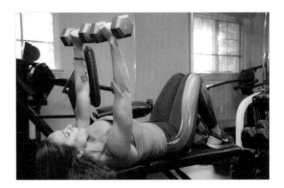

Chest Presses: Lie on a flat bench with a dumbbell in each hand and your feet flat on the bench. Push the dumbbells up so that your arms are directly over your shoulders and your palms are up. Lower the dumbbells down and a little to the side until your elbows are slightly below your shoulders. Aim to do 3 sets of 12–15 reps.

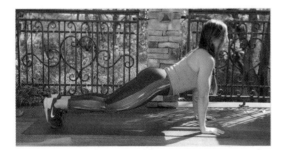
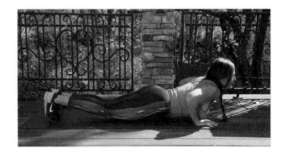

Push-ups: Start in plank position, shoulders in line with wrists, and lower your body down to the floor, keeping movements slow and controlled. Then push yourself up to starting position. Repeat until you can no longer hold your form or lift yourself off the floor. If you can't do these, it's okay to do the "girly" version where your knees are touching the floor instead! The most important thing is proper form.

IS UNDERWIRE DOING US MORE HARM THAN GOOD?

There has been a debate over potential "harmful" effects of underwire in bras for decades. In fact, according to an essay on www.bigbra.com, in two books (one written in 2002 called *Women's Bodies, Women's Wisdom*, and one in 1999 called *What Your Doctor May Not Tell You About Premenopause*) women are encouraged to stop wearing underwire bras altogether. Both cite the circulation of blood and lymph fluid around the breasts and surrounding tissue, stating that underwire puts pressure on these glands, preventing the draining of toxins from the breast.

As logical as it may sound, there has been no evidence to actually support that wearing an underwire bra is harmful—short of being a little painful if your cup size is too small (if your underwire sits in the middle of your breast instead of in the fold, it can pinch the breast tissue). If the underwire is so tight against your skin that it causes sweating underneath or so loose that it shifts and rubs, it could potentially cause or worsen skin irritations, so be conscious of that. Otherwise, go ahead and push those puppies up!

Schulman states that there is no scientific evidence that bras have any bearing at all on whether our breasts sag. In fact, Pancholi says, if anything bras can *help* in our battle against sagging. "Bras play a huge role in *preventing* sagging. The more support breasts have, the less role gravity plays over time."

A study released in 2013 made headlines around the world when it supposedly revealed that wearing a bra actually *causes* sagging because it "weakens" the muscles that hold up our breasts. Researchers in France studied a few hundred women over a fifteen-year period and measured changes in the women's breasts. They claimed that the women who never wore bras had nipples on average seven millimeters higher in relation to their shoulders than regular bra wearers. But I found a few issues with this study—the first being the relatively small sample size.

Also, other factors that we know contribute to sagging, such as genetics, number of pregnancies a woman has had, and whether or not she breastfed, were not studied.

Breast sagging is inevitable for most women, except for those with very small breasts. For women with large breasts, it could happen sooner for you because you have more weight pulling the breasts downward. But genetics can also play a part. "Some women simply tend to develop more sagging than others do, which is simply hereditary," says Orange County, California, plastic surgeon Dr. John Di Saia. Di Saia points to weight fluctuation as a factor as well: "Extreme weight loss or gain over time can also speed up [the sagging] process."

As for solutions to sagging, most experts feel that, short of surgery, the only way to prevent at least the appearance of droopiness is a good underwire push-up bra.

137

Now that we've separated the myths from the facts, let's focus on faux pas. There are plenty of them out there when it comes to bras. Want to keep your faux pas under wraps? Read on to find out how!

seven

Bra Faux Pas

and How to Fix Them

Faux pas: a false step; a mistake or wrong measure.
—Webster's Revised Unabridged Dictionary

We've all heard the term "fashion faux pas." They happen all the time. Whether it's an inadvertently exposed nipple by a celebrity on the red carpet, or a woman who simply wears an outfit that's inappropriate for the office, faux pas, or fashion mistakes, whether accidental or not, are something we often live to regret.

But when it comes to bras, what constitutes a faux pas, and how can they be avoided? Is it a strap slipping out from underneath a blouse? Is it a white bra that's glaringly obvious underneath a white top? Or perhaps it's a nipple that's popping *through* your blouse, for the entire world to see?

Celebrities know all about bra faux pas. The list of famous fashion "oops" moments involving improperly fitting undergarments (or lack thereof) is endless. Actress Tara Reid inadvertently exposed her breast while on the red carpet in 2004. In addition to her infamous pantyless peek-a-boo moment, singer Britney Spears has had many a nipple-slip, during dance rehearsals, nights out on the town, and even reportedly at a concert in 2007. Janet Jackson introduced the term "wardrobe malfunction" to the world and showed a lot more than she planned during the Super Bowl halftime show on national television in 2004, when her breast suddenly flashed across the screen and stunned the nation. Lindsay Lohan has been photographed spilling out of her top on several occasions. So have Lil' Kim, Rihanna, Lady GaGa—the list goes on. And the phenomenon is far from new—actress Jayne Mansfield reportedly exposed her breasts *intentionally* on several occasions as a way to garner publicity in the 1950s, and many others are following her lead by doing the same today (hey, no press is bad press, right?).

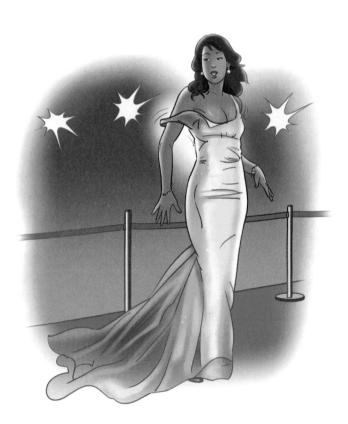

I'VE GOT 99 BRA-BLEMS BUT A NIP-SLIP AIN'T ONE

Whether you call it a wardrobe malfunction or simply a nipple slip-up, many are instances of a woman wearing the wrong bra (although Jackson's incident is still up for debate). And as these incidents show, this kind of thing happens to the best of us—even those with million-dollar paychecks and personal stylists.

So what can you do to avert your own "wardrobe malfunctions" when it comes to bras? This chapter outlines ten common "bra pas" and how to make sure they don't happen to you. Consider these your ten commandments. If you follow them, your bra faux pas will be a thing of the past.

Faux Pas #1: Slippery Straps

Problem: Your bra straps keep slipping down your shoulders or peeking out from under your tops, especially sleeveless, halter, and boat neck shirts and dresses.

"Ugly Bra Strap Syndrome is a condition that affects women around the country who let their dingy, discolored bra straps peek through their clothing," says BraStraps.com spokesperson Michelle Soudry. "Women need to realize that bra straps have an expiration date and exposing discolored or worn straps underneath a sleeveless tank is a major don't!"

Straps have long been banished to underneath blouses—or replaced, with the "invisible" clear plastic version. They don't have to be—it's OK to let your straps show when they perfectly match or coordinate with your top. "We like to think of bra straps as an extension of your fashion closet," says Soudry. "Straps essentially become a part of your outfit, for better or for worse."

Still, if you don't want your straps to show, what can you do?

Solution: First and foremost, you can simply opt for a strapless bra, or try the aforementioned clear plastic bra straps, which can be attached to any bra that has removable straps. Many convertible bras even come with a set of clear plastic straps for exactly this purpose, although I personally am not a huge fan of them, as they can look tacky. My advice? I'm with Soudry: Make your straps a part of your outfit, like an accessory!

Another alternative is to apply some double-sided tape between the straps and shirt fabric to keep them in place and in line with your top, or to use a product like Fashion Forms' Strap Tamers, which clip on to your clothes to keep slipping straps at

BRA FAUX PAS FAST FACT

According to a survey in the UK by Wonderbra, having visible bra straps is one of the worst fashion faux pas you can make. In fact, a third of women surveyed said it looks "cheap" and even men said it's a turn-off! More than half of women said it's the summer's worst style crime and will go to all lengths to avoid it, including tucking straps into their tops, going bra-less altogether, and using bikini tops instead of their bras.

bay. They work for everything from evening gowns to workout wear!

You can also look for a strap connector that links your bra straps in the back and pulls them as far inward as necessary, forming a racerback shape, to keep them out of sight.

And remember, you can always choose to show off those straps (and sex-ify those shoulders) with a decorative pair that acts as an accessory. (The only exception to this is a halter-top or an off-the-shoulder top, both of which look best with completely bare shoulders and therefore should only be worn with a strapless or halter-style bra where the strap is hidden.

145

Faux Pas #2: Peek-a-Boo Bra

Problem: Your bra is peeking out above a low neckline or at the arm openings.

Sometimes this is done on purpose—think a blouse only buttoned up halfway in order to display the bra underneath it. But unless you're Madonna, this is tough to pull off. There is a reason why bras are called *under*garments!

If you're daring and it's the right occasion, though, you might be able to let your bra *slightly* peek-through. It can be sexy if it's done *tastefully*. But sexy can turn skanky super fast if you attempt a peek-a-boo bra for an inappropriate occasion. It's NEVER appropriate for the office, the PTA meeting, or anywhere else there are impressionable *or* influential people around.

Solution: If you don't want your bra to inadvertently show, use double-sided tape to adhere it to your top in places where it could pop out. If you plan to wear a button-down shirt with a few buttons undone or another low-cut top, add a camisole underneath. And if you do want your bra to tastefully peek out (say, on an evening out), then make sure it's a beautiful lace one.

Faux Pas #3: Show-Through Bra

Problem: You can see the outline (and/or color) of your bra through your top.

Sure, sometimes you might want this to happen, like on a night out when it's part of your outfit. Usually, though, when others are able to spy your bra through your shirt, it isn't an intentional fashion choice. Wearing a dark-colored bra under a light-colored or thin top often results in this kind of a see-through situation, but the most common culprit is wearing a white bra under a white top. Logic tells you that white goes under white, but it doesn't actually work that way. And while we attest in this book that nude goes with nearly everything, the most important part is that "nearly"—there are cases in which even nude is noticeable. A very sheer black sweater, for example, or one that has an open knit, frequently displays the outline of a nude bra.

Solution: Invest in nude bras and a couple of black ones (for those sheer black tops mentioned above). To be perfectly honest, including white bras in your rotation is completely optional. Nude bras will remain fairly inconspicuous under nearly everything in your closet, whereas white ones will often show through. When you're dealing with a sheer top or dress, whether it's white, purple, or green, for the most part a nude bra is your best bet.

147

Faux Pas #4: Uniboob

Problem: Your breasts are being flattened to your chest, creating the appearance of a single mass, or "uniboob."

This is a common issue when wearing compression-style sports bras that do not have separate cups, but it can also occur when your top or dress is too tight in the chest.

Solution: If your sports bra is to blame, the best option here is to simply switch to an encapsulation-style that supports the breasts separately.

In the case of a too-tight dress or top, obviously the best option is to switch to a dress that fits well up top! But if you can't, try switching to a front-closure bra that will pull your breasts inward or adding inserts, like cutlets, that will help boost your breasts up. The cleavage created will dispel the uniboob illusion.

Faux Pas #5: Double-Bubble Booby

Problem: Your breasts are being squished in a way that creates the illusion of four boobs, or a "double-bubble," beneath your clothes.

Usually this happens when your bra is too tight, which squeezes your breast tissue up and out over the top of the cup.

Solution: Go get fitted, and make sure you aren't wearing a cup size that's too small! Another potential solution: Try a fuller-coverage bra, which will encase more of your breast tissue in the cup and leave less to bulge out of the top!

Faux Pas #6: Bra Bulge

Problem: Your breast tissue or other flesh is bulging around your bra's cups or band and is visible under or above clothing.

No one wants back bulges rippling through their sheer shirts or breast tissue billowing out underneath their underarms. Not only does this ruin the line of your clothes and create the appearance of extra weight; depending on what's causing it, it can also be uncomfortable for you.

Solution: A too-tight bra is often to blame here, so loosening your bra band a notch could help. In the case of side bulge, try switching to a front-close bra that pulls your breasts inward. This should help keep spillage to a minimum. Another option?

150

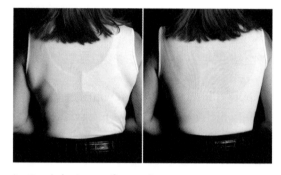

Left: Without Sassybax
Right: With Sassybax

Look for a bra where the cups come up higher on the sides. In the case of back bulge, if loosening your bra doesn't help, look for a "back smoothing" bra with a wider band.

Faux Pas #7: Nipple Poke

Problem: Your nipples are visibly "poking through" your bra and clothing.

This faux pas, also known as visible nipple syndrome, or VNS, occurs frequently enough that the subject has even been studied. Lycra brand asked women in England how they felt about nipple protrusion and a whopping 90 percent of Brits just said no to visible nips. But this can be harder for some women than for others—women with larger nipples may need a little extra help keeping theirs under wraps.

Solution: A lightly padded or lined bra will usually help you avoid showing through thin clothing. But not all dresses or tops accommodate a bra, of course, even with all the options out there. In cases like this,

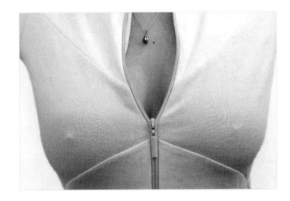

151

the best thing you can do is cover up those nips with "breast petals," which adhere to the skin on and around your nipples and can be gently peeled off when you are finished. They're also great for wearing under very sheer or non-padded bras, and work under swimsuits, too.

Another good tip? Always carry a jacket or wrap to make sure you never get cold (the biggest culprit in visible nipples).

Faux Pas #8: Braless

Problem: You are boycotting bras, and people can tell!

Women went braless for centuries . . . and in some countries still do. Believe it or not, in 2016, Hollywood celebrities like Kendall Jenner are doing it on the daily! But our better judgment (and advancements in medical science) tells us that there is a reason most women *today* don't leave the house without one on. Letting the ladies hang at all times is not recommended in either the fashion or the medical world. Despite this, a select few still opt to be bra-free.

Sometimes going commando on top is *necessary*, because of the cut of a dress or top. But even if you don't need a bra for support, concealing your nipples is simply more acceptable in society.

Solution: For gals who prefer to go braless (Whoopi Goldberg reportedly

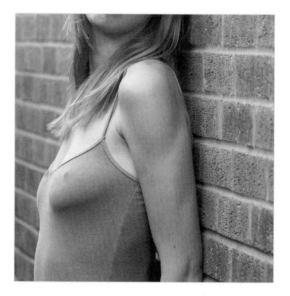

did until the age of fifty-one!), there are comfortable options available that cover up and support without constricting you. You can try a silicone adhesive bra, which is simply a pair of individual cups that adhere to your breasts, with no straps, band, or underwire to irritate you.

They are also virtually invisible under t-shirts or any other item of clothing.

You can also look for a camisole with an attached "shelf bra," which has support built in, or a bralette, which is a comfy first step in the right bra-wearing direction.

Bra-llelujah! by Spanx, the Genie Bra, and the Ahh Bra by Rhonda Shear, are all popular versions of a hosiery-style comfort bra that is perfect for easing anti-bra gals into the bra-wearing world.

153

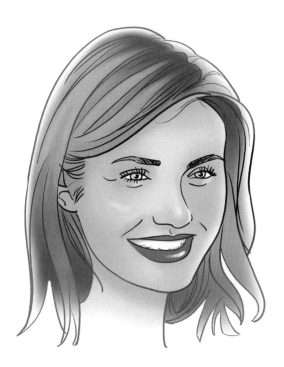

"People think I'm trying to make a fashion statement because I never wear a bra. It's really that I'm a tomboy at heart."
—Cameron Diaz

Faux Pas #9: Sagging Strapless

Problem: The evening's just begun, and your strapless bra is already heading south.

Most strapless bras use strips of silicone around the band to help it adhere to your skin. But even if you're wearing the right size, sweat, oily skin, or repeated washings can make the silicone stop sticking and start sliding.

Solution: If you don't want to toss a bra that's starting to slip altogether, you can try tightening the band, or switching to a smaller band size (which is generally recommended with strapless bras). It may be a bit uncomfortable, but at least it'll stay up. If that fails, take out your handy-dandy double-sided tape and apply it around the band for added sticking power. And you can also try backless strapless bras (also known as adhesive bras), which are sold at most department and specialty stores. Their sticky, glue-like lining adheres the cups to your skin so they stay up on their own (although dancing and subsequently sweating the night away may cause them to lose a little bit of their sticking power).

154

Faux Pas #10: Too Much Cleavage

Problem: Your low-cut top has left you a little exposed, and everyone's looking at your chest, not your face.

Cleavage is great—when it's the right amount. There *is* such a thing as "classy cleavage," but the distinction between "classy" and "trashy" can be as little as an inch too much skin. If everyone is staring, chances are you're baring a little too much boob. (*Author's note:* Feel free to skip my advice if you like the attention and the references to Pamela Anderson. I won't be insulted.)

You want to show off your best assets, but without showing it all. First and foremost, listen to your gut when you look in the mirror. If it's telling you you're showing a little too much, you probably are. (Second to my gut is my partner, who has no qualms about telling me to "put those puppies back in.")

Keep this in mind as a general rule of thumb—décolletage and the sides of your breasts can be sexy when bared, but if you're in danger of showing areola or nipple, you've gone too far.

Solution: Some bras, like padded or push-up bras, are meant to enhance cleavage, so you may want to avoid those altogether if you fear your dress or top risks showing too much. If your top has a plunging neckline, you can try adding a tissue-thin nude-colored camisole—it'll cover up some of that cleavage without ruining the look of your top.

If you're worried about your top slipping and exposing too much, you also may want to reach for the double-sided tape. Just one piece can mean all the difference between too low-cut and appropriate.

155

BRA FAUX PAS FAST FACT

Double-sided tape deserves a spot in your purse right next to your lipstick, cell phone, and gum. It's handy to always have on hand in case unexpected issues arise. It not only adheres to apparel, but to skin, too, making it the quick-fix item for everything from keeping bra straps in place to hemming a too-long pants leg. Some good choices? Hollywood Fashion Tape, which comes in useful strips, and Dress & Lingerie Tapes by Fashion Forms, which comes in a handy Scotch tape-style dispenser.

Back bulge and lumps and bumps in spots they shouldn't be is why God (or, rather, the undergarment industry) invented shapewear! Shapewear can help women of all shapes and sizes create a smoother and slimmer appearance in all their clothes. Learn more in the next chapter!

eight

Shape Up
with
Shapewear

Can you imagine a world without Spanx? Back in the late '90s, Sara Blakely cut the feet off a pair of control-top pantyhose and realized she was on to something. In 2000, Oprah came calling, Hollywood caught on, and the rest, as they say, is history. Spanx became part of nearly every woman's vocabulary, known across countries and cultures as a must-have undergarment for smoothing out all those unsightly lumps and bumps. Soon, every company in the undergarment industry was scrambling to make their own versions.

Thus, the "shapewear" phenomenon was born (because Spanx was trademarked, natch). In 2012, *Women's Wear Daily* reported that the shapewear industry was worth more than $812 billion. It has been likened to "Photoshop for your body," and it's here to stay.

Recently, women have started to catch on to the fact that shapewear isn't just for those days when you're feeling a little bloated—even the trimmest figures can use smoothing under certain fabrics. And while plenty of women use shapewear under fancier dresses, many are still not using it in their everyday wardrobes. Shapewear is all about smooth lines and creating that "perfect silhouette," no matter your shape, size, or outfit. Shapewear is a woman's best-kept secret.

"There are these great things called Spanx, and they just squeeze you in. It's terrific! That's how all the Hollywood girls do it!"
—Gwyneth Paltrow

NOT YOUR GRANDMA'S GIRDLE

• •

Shapers come in many different styles and different levels of support, or "compression," depending on their fabric and construction—some can cinch you in by up to one or two dress sizes!

We talked about compression earlier in this book in relation to certain sports bras, which "compress" your breasts so that they stay in one place during exercise. The same general concept applies to shapewear, except the compression is meant for a more aesthetic purpose: to compress your body to make it appear smaller.

Some shapers are more lightweight and stretchy, intended for smoothing, whereas others are sturdier and made with heavier fabric, and are intended to suck you in. The former is known as "light compression" whereas the latter is referred to as "firm compression."

According to Bustle.com, if there's no compression level listed on the tag, check out the garment label. The higher the nylon content, the more a garment will alter your shape.

SHAPE-UP TIP

For all the solutions shapewear offers, it has always come with an annoying challenge: Women have a hard time keeping it up! The constant shapewear "roll down" is what prompted bra designer Tara Cavosie to start HookedUp Shapewear in 2013. Her shapewear product hooks onto the back of your bra, as many other shapers do, but the back band of your bra actually *overlaps* the top of the shaper in the back so there is no room for skin or bulges to show. Genius!

FRONT

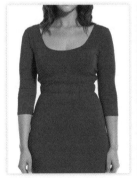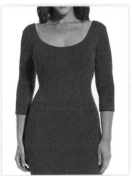

Left: Without shapewear
Right: With shapewear

BACK

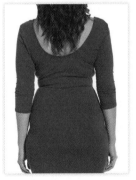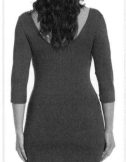

Left: Without shapewear
Right: With shapewear

TYPES OF SHAPEWEAR

· ·

SHAPING PANTIES

I like to think of these as an introductory course to shapewear. Shaping panties allow you to flatten your tummy and hips while lifting and supporting your rear, but they only go up as high as your natural waist. They can either look like a normal pair of panty briefs or go a little longer in the legs, like bike shorts, and smooth your hips, rear, and thighs. Once you try a pair of these, you will be sold on shapewear's place in your life.

HIGH-WAIST BODY SHAPERS

These pieces smooth the entire midsection, from the tummy on down through the hips (and, in some cases, thighs), as well as around the back (buh-bye, bra bulge!). They either contain a built-in bra or allow you to wear your own bra. Of those that allow you to wear your own bra, you can find styles that connect to your bra with clasps and styles with straps designed to overlap your bra.

High-waist shapers come in several styles, including a skirt or slip style, a bike short style, and a bodysuit style that does not offer thigh coverage.

THE SHAPEWEAR	WHAT IT DOES	BODY SHAPES IT'S GREAT FOR*
High-waisted Biker Short	Trims thighs and hips, firms and lifts bottom	
High-waist Slip	Firms and trims midsection and hips and defines waistline	
High-waist Bodysuit	Firms and trims midsection, defines waistline	
Shaping Panties	Firms and trims belly, hips, and bottom	

See page 89 for a refresher on your body shape!

163

FIT

· ·

It's important to get the perfect fit because, while shapewear is intended for smoothing and shaping, if it's ill-fitting, you'll end up with bulges and lumps and bumps where you didn't even have them before—kind of defeats the purpose, right? And for that, you need some measurements. The same type of tape measure we used for your bra measurements in Chapter 3 will work, but if you don't have a measuring tape, use a piece of yarn, and then measure that with a ruler.

Most shapers come in the ubiquitous S, M, and L, but they almost always offer sizing guidelines (which can differ somewhat depending on the brand), so knowing your basic measurements (bust,

SHAPE-UP TIP

Always step into your shapewear, rather than pulling it over your head. This keeps the control panels and seams in just the right position. If you have a style that hooks to your bra, such as HookedUp, connect the two *first*, leaving the bra unclasped in the back. Step into it, and then reach around and clasp your bra.

NEED A LIFT? TRY A BUTT BRA!

....

Recently, Kylie Jenner revealed on her social media accounts that it wasn't squatting at the gym (although I'm a big fan of that for boosting your booty!) or surgery that gave her that plumper, perkier, and more rounded derriere. It was shapewear! The reality star attests to her Spanx's shape-shifting abilities to take her booty from flat to Kardashian in a flash.

But if Spanx alone isn't enough to boost your booty, you can always try a butt bra! Bubbles Bodywear offers a compression garment with supportive shapers on the thighs and cutouts over your booty cheeks, so it is designed to give your derriere a lifted appearance. Or, you can opt for a padded pair of shapewear like Booty Pop!

Go ahead, fake it. We won't tell!

THE RIGHT FOUNDATION FOR YOUR FASHION

OUTFIT	THE GOAL	THE SHAPEWEAR SOLUTION
Tailored pants and top	To fight muffin top and to slim the hips and thighs	
Skinny jeans	To fight muffin top	
Gown or dress	To slim the midsection, define the waistline, and slim the hips	
Form-fitting mini dress	To slim the midsection and define the waistline	
Jumpsuit	All-over slimming	

166

waist, and hips) will help you get the best fit. For the bust measurement, wrap the tape measure around your rib cage just below your bust, as you did in Chapter 3. If the shaper you are shopping for has a built-in bra, follow the instructions for measuring your bra size, and make sure that fits correctly as well. For the waist measurement, wrap the tape measure around the narrowest part of your waist. For the hip measurement, wrap it around the fullest part of your hips.

Finally, an important tip: Don't size down! Many women mistakenly buy a SMALLER size thinking it'll cinch them in even more, only to learn that a too-small shaper just squeezes you in all the wrong places. Stick to your size!

SHAPE-UP TIP

One thing that always scares women about trying shapewear is that it can be tough to get on and off, making bathroom trips daunting. Look for a shaper that contains an opening in the crotch for easy bathroom access. Since most shapers are meant to be worn commando—why risk lines when lines are what you are trying to prevent?—all you have to do to pee is slide the fabric over, no garment removal necessary!

Now that you've gotten the skinny on shapewear, read on for swimwear tips and why bra-sized is best!

nine

Swim Support

I HEAR AS MANY COMPLAINTS FROM WOMEN ABOUT SHOPPING FOR SWIMSUITS as I do about bras. And every spring, I talk about how to find the "right" bathing suit for your shape on shows like *TODAY*, *The Meredith Vieira Show*, *The Wendy Williams Show*, and more. The reason all these shows book me for this topic year after year? Because it's just so darned hard for women to find the perfect bathing suit. First you have to find a style that you feel comfortable in, then you have to make sure it fits!

The best tip I've learned when it comes to shopping for swimwear? Buy bra-sized!

Many swimwear lines offer tops based on actual bra sizes. But even better? Many come with actual built-in bras—underwire and all! If you are a busty woman who needs a lot of support, this is the perfect (and really, as far as I'm concerned, only) option for you. Unless you want to grab that triangle top and be popping out the bottom (not a good look, ladies!).

Also keep in mind that, just like with bras, you can choose from different kinds of straps. Some swim tops have thin spaghetti straps that tie, while others have bra-like straps that you can even adjust. You can also find halter-style tops (a flattering look for larger busts) and sometimes sports bra–style racer backs, both of which add extra support.

The Swimwear Guide

ONE PIECES

Tank with built-in bra

Often has underwire for support
Often has adjustable straps

Dress

Underwire for support
Often has adjustable straps
Provides maximum rear, hip, and thigh coverage

TOPS

Padded foam triangle
bikini top

Light foam padding for shaping

Bandeau-style top

Light foam padding for shaping
Wider back for smoothing and support
Removable and adjustable straps
Boosts smaller busts

Tankini top with
built-in bra

Underwire for support
Often has adjustable straps

Corset-style top

Underwire and boning for support
Lacing for adjustability
Boosts smaller busts

BOTTOMS

Full coverage Provides full rear coverage

Moderate coverage Provides moderate rear coverage (some rear end is exposed on each side)

Brazilian Provides only slightly more rear coverage than a thong (most of the rear end is exposed)

Scrunch Provides only slightly more rear coverage than a thong (most of the rear end is exposed)

Side tie Ties at the sides for adjustability

French cut Higher leg openings lengthen the appearance of the leg

High-waisted or retro style Higher waist provides more midsection coverage

Boy cut Provides more hip, rear, and thigh coverage

Skirt Often adjustable or available in different lengths. Provides maximum rear, hip, and thigh coverage

173

SWIMWEAR SHOPPING FOR YOUR SHAPE

Don't just shop based on your bust—choose your swimsuit based on what will most flatter your figure! Follow the guide below to shop for swimwear based on your body shape and/or figure goals.

BODY SHAPE*	GOAL	LOOK FOR
Apple/ inverted triangle	Create a waistline and trim midsection Lengthen legs	Tanks with side cutouts Retro high-waisted bottoms with high-cut leg openings
Pear	De-emphasize your bottom half by drawing attention to your top half	One-shouldered styles Print or embellishment on top paired with a solid color on the bottom
Banana/rectangle	Create curves	Ruffles, embellishment, and/or padding up top Skirted or printed bottoms

See page 89 for a refresher on your body shape!

GIVING THE SWIMWEAR MARKET A BOOST

. . . .

In spring of 2015, I teamed up with swimwear designer Julie Joa for my own collection of bra-sized swimwear called The Gravity Defying Collection by Jené Luciani. We designed a bikini-style top, a corset-style top, a tankini top, and a one piece, all with built-in bras. The bikini style has thin foam padding for shaping and a band at the bottom of the cups for support, plus an adjustable T-back for even more support. The corset-style top has underwire and a lace-up back for adjustability and support, and the tankini and one piece both have underwire and adjustable bra-like straps as well. Basically, all the elements you'd find in a bra, but in a swimsuit! See the collection at JulieJoaSwim.com.

ten

Mountains

vs.

Molehills

"In junior high, a boy poured water down my shirt and yelled, 'Now maybe they'll grow.'"
– Pamela Anderson

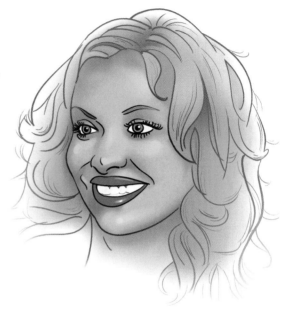

LET'S FACE IT, EVERYONE HAS PROBLEMS. FOR MANY WOMEN, THEIR BIGGEST problem weighs heavy on their chests—literally. Or perhaps not heavy enough. Whether you feel your breasts are too large or too small, there are problems you face on a regular basis—especially when it comes to bras! Luckily, there are also solutions.

MOUNTAINS

Given the emphasis our culture puts on large breasts, you'd think having them would be easy, right? Not so! The first challenge facing women with larger busts is finding bras large enough to fit. Most retailers only carry up to a DD, and if you are an "odd" size—if you have a band smaller than a 34 but a larger cup—it's even tougher finding your size in stores. Often, online shopping sites offer a larger range of sizes than department stores and chain retailers. But ordering online can be a risky and expensive proposition, since you can't try before you buy.

The websites BareNecessities.com and HerRoom.com both carry an extensive array of sizes and have great return policies, and there are also plenty of bra lines made especially for bustier gals.

Even if the larger-chested woman can find a bra in her size at the department store, she often faces an aesthetic challenge—ugly bras. Lisa Guarini, inventor of the Bra Smart (a bra mold that allows you to air dry your bras while still maintaining their shape) and self-proclaimed busty gal, has struggled with finding pretty bras her entire life. "Being a bustier woman, it has always been hard to find the right bras that fit me properly yet were stylish at the same time," says Guarini. Even while working as a bra specialist for

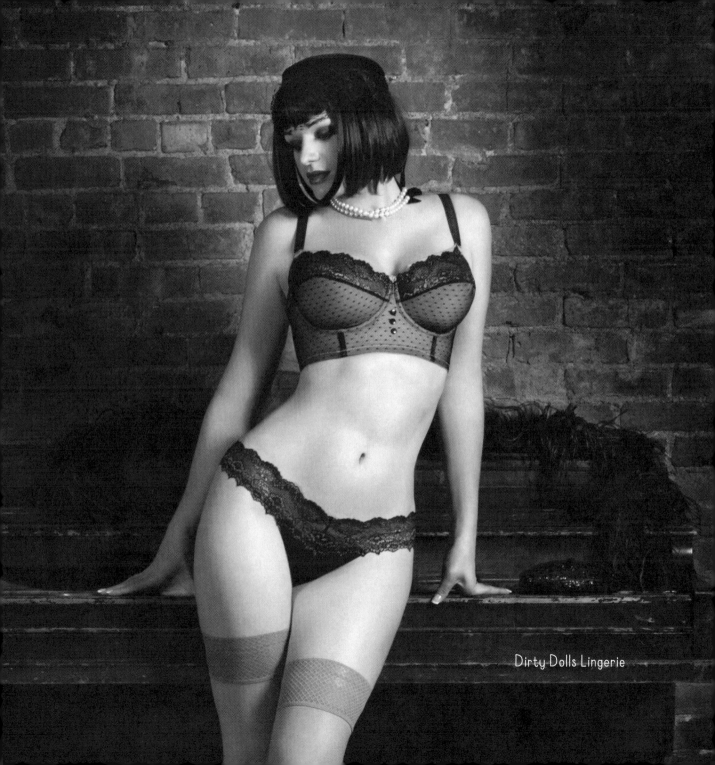

Dirty Dolls Lingerie

SUPPORTING MOUNTAINS: SPORTS BRAS

While even everyday bras are an issue, well-endowed women also have trouble when it comes to sports bras. For some larger-busted women, any form of exercise can be problematic. Many feel the need to wear two sports bras at a time to give them the proper support. While the bra industry is still struggling to come up with the perfect sports bra for the bustier athlete (during a recent trip into a Nike store where, at a 34DD, even the extra-large sports bra didn't fit me, I learned even sports apparel industry forerunners aren't keeping up with us busty gals), there are some on the market that you can try. The ENELL SPORTS Bra was specifically designed for women who are larger-busted (or are pregnant, nursing, or healing from breast augmentation surgery). It comes in ten sizes and combines the technology of both compression and encapsulation sports bra styles to make the best bra possible for women who need a little more support. Check www.enell.com for ordering options.

lingerie chain Victoria's Secret, she still felt a lack of options. "Why is it the bras for bustier women always look like granny bras?" she asks.

While you can often find prettier styles for larger sizes online, locating brick and mortar where you can try them on first is another story. Frances Crespo founded her Virginia bra-fitting salon The Full Cup in response to her years of searching for pretty bras for fuller women like herself. Her store specializes in lingerie for women who wear band sizes 28 through 48 and cup sizes C through K.

COULD YOU BE A MOUNTAIN AND NOT KNOW IT?

While most of us generally know whether we are large- or small-breasted, or somewhere in between, many women confuse the sizing system—especially cup size—with preconceived notions of what those sizes *should* look like. Here's something you should know: When it comes to bra sizes, you are often "smaller" in one measurement and "larger" in the other than you think. Let me explain.

Recently, I had a bra-fitting party at my house. Out of the fifteen or so women of all ages, shapes, and sizes that were fitted, *every single one* was wearing the wrong bra size. Another thing they all shared? All of the women were wearing a band size that was too big—and a cup size that was too small. One woman had been wearing a 38C for years. Her real size? A 30E!

While some claim that women's breasts are just bigger these days than they used to be, bra experts say the real explanation for larger cup sizes is that women are simply wearing band sizes that are more true to measurement.

"I always strived to buy a comfortable, well-fitting bra," says Crespo. "Among other things, it made a huge difference in how the rest of my clothes fit and how I felt about myself. But it was frustrating. Just because I was a DD—or so I was told for years by people who weren't as trained as my staff at The Full Cup—why couldn't I feel and look as sexy as all the other girls with smaller cup sizes and a wider range of choices in the average American store? Was it too much to ask for a bit of style with that big bra? Did they have to look so . . . utilitarian? I could not understand why it was so difficult to find good bras for the 'fuller-busted woman' like me."

Armed with her family background in the bra industry (her aunt was a bra sample–maker for nearly fifty years), her sewing expertise, and previous business experience, Crespo decided to do something about it, opening up her first store in 2003 (she now has two locations in Virginia).

Larger-breasted women also face more serious challenges. Many opt to undergo breast reduction surgery because their heavy breasts are causing them physical pain. Those who don't can face lifelong back pain and neck and shoulder strain, as well as poor quality of life, because they can't even exercise like everybody else. Women with large breasts can also have to deal with chafing, sweating, rashes, and even fungal infections in the fold of skin beneath the breasts, as described in Chapter 6. Many apply deodorant or powder to the area daily before putting on their bra, and this is my favorite trick for the band of my sports bra after a sweat session at the gym!

Besides these physical challenges, larger breasts can simply have a tough time "fitting in." It's hard to find clothing that fits properly; either tops fit over the breasts but are baggy around the waist, or they fit at the waist and are too tight across the chest. And lower-cut shirts can be perilous. "Unless you want to have it all hanging out there, your obstacle is 'containing' your breasts," says Tara Cavosie, a bra designer for Fashion Forms who attests she has always been busty. "Especially during pregnancy, a larger-breasted woman will get even bigger. This is where minimizing comes in."

There are special "minimizing" bras on the market made just for more ample women that not only make you look more

SPECIAL SIZING FOR MOUNTAINS

Sizing can be confusing when it comes to larger cup sizes. A DD to some retailers can be an E to others. Here is a chart that will help explain sizes for DD and up.

DIFFERENCE BUST MEASUREMENT MINUS BAND SIZE	US CUP SIZE
5"	DD/E
6"	DDD/F
7"	G
7.5"	GG
8"	G, H
9"	H, I
10"	H, I, J
11"	HH
11.5" – 13"	I
13" – 15.5"	J
15.5" – 17"	K, JJ

proportioned, but offer extra support as well. Or if you don't want to specifically choose a minimizing bra, you can look for a regular bra that will give you the support you need. Cavosie recommends looking for the following elements:

- Full coverage cups
- Wide shoulder straps
- Underwire
- Back band material that includes stretch
- Only very thin padding or lining

On the flip-side, Cavosie says larger-busted women should avoid the following:

- Plunge or demi bras, which are made to enhance cleavage
- Very thin straps
- Sheer, thin microfiber fabrics

The wrong bra can also make top-heavy women appear heavier than they actually are. As Staci Berner, creator of the Unbelivabra by Shapeez, explained, "While I'm not extremely large breasted at a 36C, I do carry the majority of my weight on my upper body. I found that my traditional bras were making

186

"I wanted to be the first woman to burn her bra, but it would have taken the fire department four days to put it out."
– Dolly Parton

me look heavier than I was because the elastic bands were creating unnecessary back bulges and bra overhang, which I was very self conscious of. I searched for bras without the bands but none had the adequate breast support and shaping I needed." So Berner took matters into her own hands and the Unbelievabra was born. "I'm a typical woman who has had two kids, so going braless was not an option for me. The only thing I could do was create the bra of my dreams myself. We appropriately named this new invention the Unbelievabra and started selling them online and to retail stores under the company name of Shapeez. So now, women don't have to sacrifice breast support and shaping to get a totally comfortable, seamless, smooth look from front to back."

While it may be difficult for larger breasted women to find the right bra, once you do, feeling confident is key. "Bras are more than simply a foundation garment," says Guarini. "A bra reflects everything a woman is and everything she can be . . . fun and flirty, sexy and provocative,

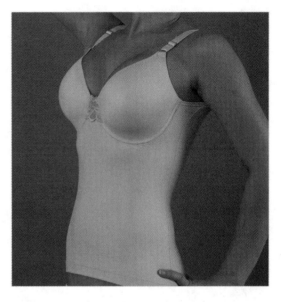

The Unbelievabra by Shapeez

187

strong and supportive. When you are wearing a great bra that gives you perfect support and makes you look good, you feel confident. And just as smaller-sized women are insecure about their chest, so are us larger ladies!"

Speaking of the smaller-busted ladies, they face an array of issues and challenges, too.

The Little Bra Company

MOLEHILLS

· ·

Ask any ample-breasted woman and she'll tell you that women with smaller breasts definitely have it easier. They can fit into almost any top. They don't have issues with exercising and don't have to worry about breast-induced back, neck, or shoulder pain. But in our breast-obsessed culture, many smaller-breasted women go under the knife to attain what their larger-busted counterparts were born with. Those who don't choose surgery rely on their bras to fill out what Mother Nature didn't provide—or at least just fit well. Unfortunately, women with smaller breasts don't seem to have any more luck than women with larger breasts!

Emily Lau started The Little Bra Company after years of frustrating trips to the lingerie stores. Lau felt that the bras that fit her small frame well looked like training bras, and the sexy ones never fit quite right. "I spent years looking ridiculous wearing ill-fitting bras. That is, until a couple of years ago when I started working with some experts to design the perfect-fitting bra for my petite body type and then tested it out on some friends."

Her yearning to make the most of her assets (without the help of saline or silicone) prompted her to make "the perfect little bra." Her bras have specially designed

ENHANCING MOLEHILLS: WANT THE ILLUSION OF MORE CLEAVAGE?

Besides wearing a bra that pushes your breasts up and together, or placing silicone inserts inside your bra to further boost breasts up, you can also dust a little shimmery bronzer between your breasts to add more "depth" to the area.

"contoured cups" that help create the illusion that smaller-breasted have more than they actually do. "I find that smaller-breasted women often resign themselves to wearing camisole bras or nothing at all," says Lau. "When I get to personally fit my customers, it's always so exciting to see their reactions. I get hugs and high-fives from women who thought they could never have cleavage. They tell me that they have never had a bra that fit the way one of mine fits and they love it because it makes them feel pretty!" Some of her bras start in as small as a 28 band size and none are larger than a B cup. Almost all are decorative and fashionable—something she says you don't often find in smaller sizes at other retailers. You can find Lau's bras online at www.herroom.com, www.brasmyth.com, www.barenecessities.com, and at www.thelittlebracompany.com.

Another company, Itty Bitty Bra (www.ittybittybra.com), has a similar mission. It offers pretty, decorative bras in sizes AA through B. Lula Lu, a petite lingerie company based in California, also specializes in hard-to-find smaller bra sizes such as AA and A cups and lingerie that flatter the smaller figure. Even though it calls itself a "petite" lingerie store, the store's founder Ellen Shing says they are not about height (the formal definition of petite in fashion is 5'4" and under), but rather frame and bust size, and have customers who are 6 feet tall.

At a 36A, Shing says she has what is considered to be an "odd" size because of her bigger back and smaller bust. Numerous bra-shopping trips left her discouraged as she couldn't find any of the styles she liked

ENHANCING MOLEHILLS:
WHY DEMIS ARE DESIGNED JUST FOR YOU

Whether you want to increase your size or just be more comfortable, demi cups are a great option for you smaller-breasted ladies because they're designed with you in mind. They have the least breast coverage but their slightly tilted cups offer a boost by pushing the breasts towards the center for increased cleavage. Demi cups are also designed with shallower/shorter underwire to prevent poking petite women.

in her size. "It's not that manufacturers don't make 36As, it's just that a lot of the stores either didn't stock them or didn't re-order after they ran out," says Shing. "I then got curious about my other friends' bra shopping experiences, as some of them have even smaller busts than I do. So I asked around and heard all kinds of stories, such as they were often told to go to the children's department even though they were grown women! So, after doing a lot more research, I decided to take the plunge and open up my store and e-commerce site, as it seemed there was a need for this."

Shing eventually launched her own bra line, Lula Lu Petites, because she couldn't find a lot of the styles or fits her customers were asking for in existing lines. Shing's line can be purchased on her website at www.lulalu.com. "I really enjoy what I do, as I feel my store and website help make a lot of small-busted women feel like, 'Ahhh, there *are* bras in my size!' rather than feeling dejected whenever they go to other lingerie stores and leave feeling like there is something wrong with them," she says.

For women who love their petite stature but sometimes want an even bigger boost, Victoria's Secret and Montelle Intimates are now making bras that claim to enlarge your breasts by up to two cup sizes.

Another challenge those who are "flat-chested" face is that they may not even register on the size chart in the first place. Bra measurements are calculated based on the assumption that women have an inch or more difference between their band size measurements and their cup size measurements. If you fall into the category of women who don't have that inch, your best option may be to go to the store and try on bras that are closest to your size, then add some cutlets to help fill it out.

MOUNTAINS VS. MOLEHILLS: BUST BUDDIES FACE OFF!

Time to look on the bright side! I consulted some friends, both large- and small-busted, and asked them to give me the pros of both! Here are their top ten lists.

Small Breasts: The Pros

1. You don't get back pain.
2. You can wear almost any shirt without the risk of looking "slutty," and you are less likely to be stereotyped in a job interview.
3. You can wear your "true size" in shirts and dresses instead of having to go a size up.
4. You can find a bikini top that doesn't expose a whole boob.
5. Lying on your belly isn't painful.
6. You don't get under-boob sweat.
7. You have less fear of saggy/droopy boobs.
8. You can go braless and still be perky, or add a push-up bra for major cleavage—the best of both worlds!
9. You can wear sexier bras instead of "granny-style" minimizers.
10. Guys always know where your eyes are.

Large Breasts: The Pros

1. They help balance out a curvy figure.
2. They create the illusion of a tiny waist.
3. They give you an excuse to deduct an extra five to ten pounds off what the scale says.
4. You "fill out" your clothes better.
5. You don't have to fear strapless dresses will fall down.
6. No risk of "false advertising." What you see is what you get!
7. You don't need to spend money on cutlets, push-up pads, or anything else—you have cleavage naturally!
8. Small-chested women are usually jealous.
9. You never risk being mistaken for a boy.
10. Men love them!

LOVING YOUR BREASTS JUST THE WAY THEY ARE

· ·

Many of us look in the mirror and see something completely different than what the rest of the world sees, and often so-called "imperfections" (such as breasts that are too large, too small, saggy, or even lopsided) can seem glaringly obvious when in reality someone else wouldn't even notice them.

Body image expert Sarah Maria (www.sarahmaria.com) says society is to blame. "As a society, we have projected certain images of beauty into the world. We then idealize these images and internalize them, believing that we should live up to some external standard of beauty. We attempt to achieve beauty by complying with some ideal, as opposed to connecting with our own inner, innate beauty. When this happens, women suffer."

Using undergarments to mold women's bodies into a desired shape or hide so-called "flaws" is nothing new. The corset of the nineteenth and twentieth centuries created coveted curves by pushing up the breasts and narrowing the waist in order to emphasis womanly breasts, hips, and derriere. And with all the options available to us today, it's easy for us to obsess over our bodies. A thin frame with large breasts is in, sending millions of us not just to the store for expensive bras and accessories, but to the gym—and the plastic surgeon's office.

While it's not always realistic to expect a woman to accept her body just the way it is, there are some steps you can take to at least be more at peace with the way you look. Maria says the first step is identifying exactly what it is that makes you think your body and your breasts are unacceptable. "Learn how to identify these thoughts and detach yourself from them. It's important to realize that thoughts have no truth to them other than the truth *you* give them. Those thoughts that make you feel bad about your body can just be disregarded and discarded."

Website www.myintimacy.com suggests, "Try to cultivate a positive attitude about your breasts and your body in general. Decide to love your breasts as they are. Ideally, your breasts will be your breasts for life. Changing your attitude is entirely in your power."

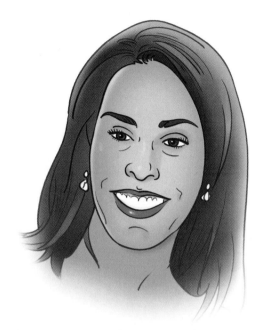

195

"You know they say beauty comes from the inside, so buy a good bra!"
– Melissa Rivers

The lesson to be learned in this chapter—and in this book—is that good things can come in both large and small packages, and the right bra can help you make the most of whatever package you've got. Bras shouldn't be a crutch, but they can be a tool—a tool you use to make yourself look and feel the best you can, from the inside out!

SHOPPING TIPS

Now that you've read *The Bra Book*, you're ready to go shopping! Here is a compilation of some of the book's top tips that you can take along with you.

1. Choose a store that has a wide selection of bras and *trained* bra fitters on hand.

2. Try to avoid bra shopping during "that time of the month." You can be up to a full cup size bigger when you're on your period!

3. Go to the store armed with a list of what you need and plan to buy: i.e., two nude bras, two black bras, one strapless, one sports bra, one bra without underwire for comfort (this will vary from person to person). Remember: nude goes under *nearly everything*.

4. Be aware of your body type so you know what bras to look for. For example, if you are more of a top-heavy "apple," you likely will be looking for fuller coverage bras, not demi-cups.

5. Wear or bring a thin t-shirt to the store so you can see what each bra looks like under the sheerest of circumstances.

6. At the store, find a bra fitter that you feel comfortable with, and get measured to find your proper size.

7. Be open-minded about your size. If you're surprised (or disappointed), remember that size is just a number (and a letter!). The proper fit of the bra is the most important part.

8. Use your size only as a *guideline*. You will still need to try the bras on!

9. If you're in a bind and there's a bra that you really love but they don't have your size, it's usually OK to go up a band size and down a cup size. For example, if you are a 34DD, try the bra in a 36D and see if it works.

10. Don't be afraid to put the bra on and face yourself in the mirror with a critical eye. If you see any gaps, spillage, digging in, or other signs of poor fit, it's not the right bra. Turn around and look at the back as well. The back band can be very telling too when it comes to proper fit.

11. Don't forget to pick up some bra accessories, too, so you avoid any faux pas! Breast petals and double-sided tape are always good to have on hand.

12. Don't get stuck in a size rut. Write down the date of your visit and be sure to plan another one six months to a year later!

CARE TIPS

Your bras are one of—if not *the*—most important articles of clothing you own. Yet when it comes to care, they often get neglected. In fact, bras are probably also the most abused, mistreated garments we own. We throw them in the washing machine unprotected, bend their underwires, misshape their cups, wear them month after month without replacement, and then curse them when they're not as comfortable or supportive as they once were.

Caring properly for your bras is important, but I know we're all busy. It's not realistic to expect every woman to take the time to hand-wash her bras. So here are some tips on caring for your bras in a way that will extend their life and keep you looking forever stylish, *without* cramping your style.

WASHING AND DRYING

We know it's best to hand-wash and soak your bras, shapewear, and swimsuits with either a gentle detergent like Woolite or a soda-based cleansing wash like Forever New. In fact, it can make your bra last up to 30 percent longer. But that doesn't mean the washing machine is the enemy. Some things to keep in mind if you're machine-washing your bras:

▶ Don't forget to check the tag. If your bra has special washing instructions, follow them.

▶ A front-loading washer is ideal; it doesn't have a drum and is therefore gentler on your clothes. However, if you don't have one of these, be sure to use a netted garment bag (some are made especially for bras) or a protective casing like the plastic ball-shaped BraBABY. Using something like the BraBABY also helps retain the shape of the bra's cups, which often end up getting crushed. When a bra is tossed in alone, without "protection," a top-loading washing machine can be especially dangerous to straps and bands, as they can "catch" on the drum and get damaged. In the case of an underwire bra, the machine can damage the underwire by bending it or weakening the fabric, causing poke-through, so you'll want to take extra care.

▶ Be sure to first fasten the hooks, so they don't catch on other garments.

▶ Never use bleach, and always use a gentle detergent.

▶ Put the machine on the gentlest cycle possible (most have a "delicate" cycle) and always use cold water. Bras are made from very sensitive fabrics and excessive heat can ruin them.

While machine-washing your bras can work if you're careful, machine-drying is NEVER okay; the heat from the dryer is especially bad for your bras! You should always hang your bras or lay them flat to dry. A good option for helping your bra retain its shape while air-drying is the Bra Smart. You just place your bra into the bra-shaped plastic mold and let it dry with the help of ventilated slits in the plastic. It even comes with a hanger for hanging.

Whatever you do, do not dry clean or iron your bras. Again, exposing your bra to heat is a bad idea!

If you're lucky enough to have a partner who does the laundry, either share these tips or put your bras aside and do them yourself. He may not "get" the importance of taking such care.

STORING

How you store your bras can also have an effect on their longevity. The best way to store bras is to lay them flat in a drawer (unhooked), one right after another. The cups of one bra can sit inside the cups of the next, with tissue paper placed in between. Never fold the cups or shove your bra into or through a too-tight space, as this can permanently damage the cups and underwire.

PACKING

Packing your bras for a trip can be especially troublesome. To avoid damaging them while travelling, place softer items like socks inside the cups to help them retain their shape, and nestle them into their own spot in your suitcase, preferably on the side where there aren't any items on top of them.

Another option: Pick up a bra-shaped case, like the Bra Bag from The Brag Company (www.thebragcompany.com). The company that makes the Bra Smart also makes a travel case that keeps your bras from being crushed in your suitcase. You can find it at www.smartbroad.com.

MORE TIPS TO EXTEND THE LIFE OF YOUR BRA

▶ Wash them frequently (if possible, after every use) to remove dirt and oil that accumulate during the day.

▶ If you don't wash your bras after every use, at the very least don't wear the same bra day after day. Instead, rotate between three or four, giving each one a day or two in-between to "rest." Contact with your body heat day after day will cause the bra to stretch and deteriorate faster.

HOW YOU KNOW IT'S TIME TO REPLACE YOUR BRA

As a rule of thumb, a bra you wear a lot will need to be replaced after approximately six months because of stretching, wear, and tear—a small price to pay for comfort and support! Here are a few indicators that it's time to give your bra the old heave-ho:

▶ You find yourself moving to the tighter hook as time passes, indicating that the fabric is starting to stretch out.

▶ The color starts to fade.

▶ The fabric starts looking worn.

▶ The underwire starts poking out.

Utilize these tips, and you and your bras will have a long and happy life together!

BRA SHOPPING TIPS FOR OUR BOYS

Lingerie buying can be one of the most romantic things a man does in a relationship. Guys, get a clue—women LOVE lingerie, or really anything that makes us feel sexy, especially if you picked it out for us!

Ladies, your man isn't a mind reader. Sometimes you just have to tell him what you really want! Believe me; he'll be grateful for the guidance. So be sure to tear out the tips below and fill out the cheat sheet on the next page to share with him—preferably before the next big holiday!

Tip 1: Don't be afraid to approach the salesperson. For many men, the lingerie store can be a scary place. Navigating aisles and aisles of silk, satin, and lace, with numbers and size configurations more complicated than a calculus class, can be more than just daunting; it can be downright frightening. But that's what the staff is there for, and believe me, they see dozens of men like you come through those doors each and every day. When I worked at Victoria's Secret in college, one of the things we were specifically taught was how to spot an uncomfortable male shopper, make him more comfortable, and help him choose the right item for his significant other.

Tip 2: Don't try to guess her size! Telling the saleswoman, "She's kinda like, um, around your size," likely won't help you figure it out. You actually might want to raid her bra drawer, read the tags, and write down what they say—or, if it's still not clear, throw a couple of them in a bag and bring them with you!

The salesperson will then have a better idea of what sizes and styles will suit your partner best.

Tip 3: Buy for her, not you! While most women do like their guy's input, we also want to wear bras and lingerie that make *us* feel pretty. Now is not the time to pressure her into the bra with the cutout nipples that she was so resistant to before. It's also obvious when a man is buying for himself—and that takes away from the specialness of such an intimate gift. It's safest to think "romantic" and not "racy." You want to impress her, not offend her. When in doubt, a bra and panty set is rarely a bad idea—a survey by Uplifted (www.upliftedlingerie.co.uk) showed that 60 percent of women like their lingerie gifts in sets!

Tip 4: Don't go it alone. If you're close to her best friend or sister, you can always consult them for advice. Make a list of their suggestions and bring that list with you to the store . . . or even better, bring her friend or sister, and let them help you pick something out.

Tip 5: Don't forget to keep the receipt in case she wants (or needs) to return or exchange. It's hard to buy for another person, especially when it comes to clothing. This way if it doesn't fit or she doesn't quite like the way the *style* fits her, she can return it. You shouldn't take it as an insult to your manhood; sometimes she just knows what she likes best!

Tip 6: If you're really unsure, why not let *her* choose what she wants and then just provide the cash? But that's only if you've exhausted all other options. She'll be proud of you if you give it a go on your own first!

BRA SHOPPING CHEAT SHEET

My bra size is _____

My measurements are:

Bust _____

Waist _____

Hips _____

·········· (SELECT ONE) ··········

I prefer:
- ○ fuller coverage
- ○ demi cup

I like my bras to:
- ○ minimize my breast size
- ○ maximize my breast size
- ○ give me lots of support

·········· (CIRCLE ONE) ··········

I like padding .... or .... I don't like padding

I like my bras with embellishments .. or .... I like my bras plain

I like matching panties .... or .... I don't really care

My favorite bras are:

Backless strapless   Strapless   Balconette   Bandeau   Bralette

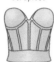

Bustier/Corset   Convertible   Demi-cup   Front-closure   Full-coverage

Minimizer   Padded   Plunge   Racerback   Sports

T-shirt   Other _____

My favorite bra colors are:

Other _____

My favorite materials are:

 Cotton   Lace   Satin    Silk   Other _____

I feel sexiest in _____

Don't even bother buying me _____

PHOTO CREDITS

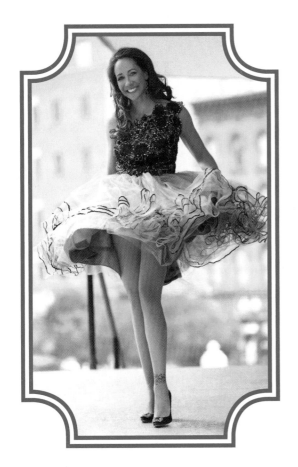

Hailed as a "brilliant bra guru" by BRAVO-TV, "the country's foremost authority on all things bras" by Dr. Oz, and a "stylist extraordinaire" and "bra fit guru" by the *New York Daily News* and *Woman's World Magazine*, Jené Luciani is a nationally acclaimed fashion journalist, lifestyle expert, tastemaker, TV personality, spokesperson, and author. She hosted Lifetime Network's *Mom's Personal Shopper* series on the Lifetime Moms channel, and she appears regularly on NBC's *TODAY*, *The Wendy Williams Show*, *Dr. Oz*, and *The Meredith Vieira Show*, among others. She has hundreds of published bylines to her name in publications such as *SHAPE* and the *Huffington Post*. Besides *The Bra Book*, she is the co-author with Jacqueline Laurita of *Get It! A Beauty, Style and Wellness Guide to Getting Your "It" Together* (BenBella Books, 2016).

When she's not appearing on TV or giving advice in print, Jené swaps her heels for sweats as a busy mom leading a "quiet life" in upstate New York with her boyfriend and children, while also enjoying serving as mistress-of-ceremonies for and on the committees of numerous philanthropic causes. You can find out more about her by visiting her online at JeneLuciani.com.

Want More on Bras and *The Bra Book?*

· ·

Then be sure to visit www.thegetitmom.com. The site is chock-full of info you won't find in the book, Jené's "picks" and where to find them online, plus articles and more! It's a wealth of bra and style information that you'll only find online!

Also be sure to look for *The Bra Book* fan page on Facebook and follow Jené on Twitter at @jeneluciani and on Instagram at @jeneontv.

COLOPHON

This book and cover were created in Adobe InDesign by Kit Sweeney. Cover illustrations and most other interior illustrations were drawn by Ralph Voltz. Text is set in Adobe Garamond Pro, with accents in Catalina Clemente, Sofia Pro, and Bickham Script Pro. The book was printed by Versa Press.

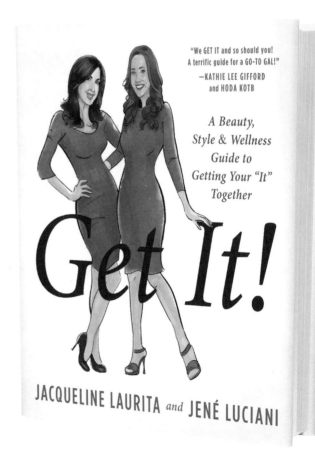